To David Webb
with thanks and best
wishes
Michael Lee
November
2003.

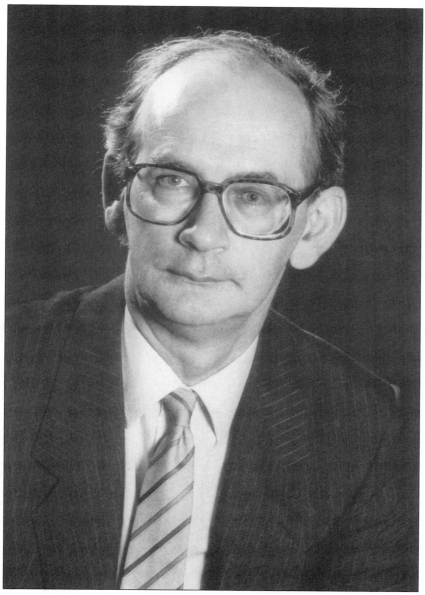

The author, aged 60, shortly before retirement.

Stood on the
Shoulders of Giants

Stood on the Shoulders of Giants
A Medical Odyssey

by

MICHAEL RADCLIFFE LEE
MA DM DPhil (Oxon) FRCP FRCPE FRSE

Emeritus Professor of Clinical Pharmacology
and Therapeutics
University of Edinburgh

One Time Somerset Thornhill Scholar of
Brasenose College, Oxford and Beit Memorial
Fellow for Medical Research

The Memoir Club

© Michael Radcliffe Lee 2003

First published in 2003 by
The Memoir Club
Whitworth Hall
Spennymoor
County Durham

British Library Cataloguing in
Publication Data.
A catalogue record for this book
is available from the
British Library.

ISBN: 1 84104 078 9

Typeset by George Wishart & Associates, Whitley Bay.
Printed by CPI Bath

Pigmaei gigantum humeris impositi
plusquam ipsi gigantes vident.

Pigmies placed on the shoulders of giants
see more than the giants themselves.

Didacus Stella
Lucan 10 Volume 2
2nd Century A.D.

Preface

He who has begun has half done.
Have the courage to be wise.
Horace 65-8 BC
Epistles I ii 40.

THE QUESTION arises straightaway. Why write a memoir? Of course it is a measure of vanity, and ego satisfying, that anyone would want to publish your ramblings, and it would be even more flattering if anyone might wish to purchase and read them! To the potential purchaser I would say at once that this is not in the usual run of biographies. I have tried to convey a sense of my struggle against both circumstances and illness. It has not been unalloyed joy. There have been conflicts, delays and disappointments along the way, many resulting from my own deficiencies and some being thrust upon me by others. I have also attempted to convey the venal organization of Medicine in the 1960s, some of which spilled over into problems in the 1990s. These deficiencies should have been tackled earlier but as Lord Acton said, 'Power tends to corrupt and absolute power to corrupt absolutely'. For too long Medicine was a cosy secret society!

The life I have pursued for the last forty years was arduous. In particular the demands of academic medicine with teaching, research, clinical work and administration were, at times, intolerable. The financial rewards could not match those of private practice. As a result, as I write recruitment to Academic Medicine has fallen away badly and many posts remain unfilled. I hope to show in this odyssey that this enterprise is an honourable one, worthwhile in its own right, whatever the outside world may think or say of it.

In the course of my voyage, I ran across a number of giants who, at various times, helped, stimulated and irritated me. These heroes became, in one way or another, role models. Often they taught me what I should aspire to be and on occasion what I should try to avoid! For good or ill, they influenced my developing career extensively, until at last I felt able to direct a small research group of my own. I also talk frankly of disappointments and difficult relationships both in London and at Leeds. Many medical memoirs are anodyne and, not to put too fine a point on it, somewhat dull. I hope therefore to convey some sense of the excitement of basic and clinical research; its highs and lows; the successes and failures. Indeed an alternative title I considered seriously for this memoir was 'Riding the Rollercoaster'. I trust that this honest no holds barred account of my professional life will stimulate others to pursue the difficult path of the clinical scientist, lying as it does on the margins between clinical medicine and laboratory investigation.

Finally two disclaimers. First I have dispensed with the usual foreword by a colleague, as in my experience, they usually end up as a sycophantic encomium, despite their best intentions. Second, many people have helped me along the way and I hope most of them have been acknowledged in the body of the text. Nevertheless, some will have been omitted inadvertently. For this I apologize and ask them to take their reward from the second part of this quotation from Ecclesiastes Chapter 44, which refers to unsung heroes and heroines.

> Let us now praise famous men and our fathers that begat us. Leaders of the people by their counsels and by their knowledge of learning, wise and eloquent in their instruction. And some there be which have no memorial but these were merciful men whose righteousness hath not been forgotten.

I will leave the reader to judge how well I have achieved these disparate objectives. The least I can hope for is they will not be bored!

Contents

Illustrations

Short Curriculum Vitae

1934 Born Manchester, England, 21 November.

1939 September
War with Germany declared whilst in Isle of Man.

1940 January
Entered Victoria Avenue Primary School, Higher Blackley.

1941 November
Primary School bombed.
Contracted rheumatic fever for second time.

1942 November
Slate injury to right eye.

1945 May
Victory in Europe Day.

1945 August
Victory against Japan Day while returning from the Isle of Man.

1946 January to March
Entered for eleven plus; Manchester Grammar School and William
Hulme's School.

1946 September
Entered Sale High School for Boys Preparatory School for
Manchester Grammar School.

1947 Mother slowly developing pernicious anaemia. Delay in diagnosis.

1948 September
Transferred from Sale High to Manchester Grammar School (Main
School) in Rusholme off Old Hall Lane.

1950 June
Take School Certificate: six Distinctions; two Credits.
Form Prize in History.

1952   June
Higher School Certificate: three Distinctions. State Scholarship.
Meet Kathleen for the first time.

1952   November
After Examination awarded Somerset Thornhill Closed
Scholarship to Brasenose College, Oxford University.

1953   October
Entered Brasenose as a Freshman.

1956   June
Awarded First Class Honours (BA) in Animal Physiology.

1956   July
Entered Manchester University for Clinical Course. Awarded
Scholarship (Non-Stipendiary).

1959   July
Qualified BM B.Ch (Oxon) in Clinical Medicine.
Preliminary registration with General Medical Council as Medical
Practitioner.

1959   August to 1960 January
House Surgeon to Mr Hall Drake; Mr Magauran; and Mr
Macfadyean at the Royal Lancaster Infirmary. Meet Judith Ann
Horrocks SRN.

1960   February to July
House Physician to Professor D.A.K. Black at the Manchester
Royal Infirmary.

1960   August 27
Married to Judith Ann Horrocks at Southey Street Methodist
Church, Keswick, Cumberland.

1960   August to 1961 May
Senior House Officer in Medicine to the Pneumoconiosis
Research Unit of the Medical Research Council at Llandough
Hospital, Cardiff (Dr J. Gilson, Director).

1961   April
Took and passed the Membership Examination of the Royal
College of Physicians of London.

1961   May to 1969 January
        In the Regius Professor of Medicine's Unit at Oxford University
        (Sir George Pickering, Director). Successively as Junior Lecturer;
        Beit Memorial Fellow and Full Lecturer.

1962   December
        Stephen Michael Lee born.

1965   March
        Karen Elizabeth Lee born.

1966   April
        Awarded Doctor of Philosophy Degree (D.Phil) for thesis entitled
        'The Estimation of Renin in Biological Fluids'.

1967   September to 1968 August
        American Heart Association Fellowship to learn the Principles of
        Radioimmunoassay with Dr J.T. Potts Jr at National Institutes of
        Health, Bethesda, Maryland, USA.

1969   February to 1971 October
        Moved to St Thomas' Hospital Medical School, London, as
        Lecturer in Medicine.

1969   May
        Published 'Renin and Hypertension; A Modern Synthesis'. Lloyd-
        Luke Publications, London.

1970   May
        Awarded Doctor of Medicine Degree (DM Oxon) on basis of
        above publication.

1971   November until 1973 October
        Medical Director then Managing Director, Weddel
        Pharmaceuticals, West Smithfield, London EC1.

1973   November until 1984 September
        Senior Lecturer in Clinical Pharmacology and Therapeutics,
        University of Leeds, West Yorkshire.

1977   April
        Awarded Fellowship of Royal College of Physicians, London
        (FRCP).

1983 February
Developed pernicious anaemia.

1984 October until 1995 September
Professor of Clinical Pharmacology and Therapeutics, University of Edinburgh, Scotland.

1985 May
Awarded Fellowship of Royal College of Physicians of Edinburgh (FRCPE).

1990 April
Awarded Fellowship of Royal Society of Edinburgh (FRSE).

1995 October
Retired from University of Edinburgh Medical School.

1996 January to 1998 December
Advising Consultant to Astra Pharmaceuticals PLC, Beaverbank Park, Edinburgh.

1999 Up to present day
Continuing studies on Medical History, the stories and legends of medicinal and poisonous plants.

Acknowledgements

A MEMOIR SUCH AS THIS would not have come to fruition without the efforts of many people in a number of institutions.

My particular thanks go to Mrs May Gibb for her indefatigable secretarial help, often in difficult circumstances; to Dr Andrew Douglas of Edinburgh, whose Presidential address to the British Thoracic Society on Samaritanism helped to crystallize my own thoughts on the ethics of medical practice; and to the staff of the Memoir Club who helped at every step of the way.

Then to people who provided material:- The *Manchester Evening News* for the photographs of Charlie Mitten and Cyril Washbrook; the High Master, Dr Martin Stephen and the Surmaster, Mr Ian Thorpe of the Manchester Grammar School (Eric James and the school); the librarian, Ms Elizabeth Kay and the archivist, Mrs Elizabeth Boardman, of Brasenose College (for the coat of arms); the archivist, Dr James Peters, of the John Rylands Library at the University of Manchester (Picture of Sir Douglas Black); the *Western Mail*, Cardiff (Llandough hospital); Dr Valerie Anderton, together with Mr Michael Stewart, both of Lancaster, for material on the Infirmary there; and Mr Michael Horrocks for the photograph of the Pier Head at Liverpool.

The Manx National Heritage, at Douglas, kindly gave its permission to reproduce the coat of arms of the island and obtained photographs of the steamships *Mona's Isle* and *Viking*; the Liverpool Maritime Museum helped with the illustrations of the *Queen Mary* and the *Empress of Canada*.

The photograph of Smithfield Market came from the Press Association; that of Leeds General Infirmary is courtesy of the *Yorkshire Post*; and the one of the Old College at Edinburgh from Susan Halcro of the Public Affairs department of that University.

I am also grateful to the Keeper of Munk's Roll at the Royal College of Physicians of London for the obituaries (and photographs) of A.L. Cochrane and G.W. Pickering; and to the Librarian, Mr Iain Milne, and his colleagues Mr J. Dallas and Professor I. Donaldson at the Royal College of Physicians of Edinburgh for their help throughout this work and in particular with the reproductions of Death's Doings, the engraving of the University of Manchester, and the book cover. Dr Thomas Tolley of the Department of Fine Art at Edinburgh University advised on the place of the good Samaritan in medieval and modern art.

Finally there are three individuals who also deserve special mention: Mr John White of Fractal Press, Grassington, Yorkshire, who expertly repaired and restored my battered old family photographs; Mrs K.E. Clarke, my daughter, who prepared the Index; and Dr Stephen M. Lee, my son, who advised on the historical accuracy of several important points in relation to the course of the Second World War.

I should also say, in closing this section, that over the last fifty years I have worked with (and for) many colleagues both medical and scientific. They have all contributed, in some measure, to what has become the essence of this, my odyssey. I thank them.

CHAPTER 1

Beginnings:
24 Tweedale Avenue, Blackley

A man travels the world over in search of what he needs and returns home to find it.

George Moore 1852-1933
The Brook Kerith Ch. 11

FROM THE MOMENT I can first remember anything, to the time that I left home for Oxford University, the council house in Tweedale Avenue was central to my development.

Blackley was a dismal suburb of North Manchester bestriding the roads to the mill towns of Bury, Middleton and Rochdale. It was filled largely with council houses thrown up at pace in the Thirties to deal with the housing shortage. These houses were not well finished. They were draughty and damp and needed constant maintenance. Nevertheless, Harry and Jean Lee regarded them as a distinct improvement on their previous dwelling when they moved into number 24, as a newly built house in the middle of the 1930s.

At least the house had a garden at the front and side and also a 'coal hole' where the coalman delivered his sacks once a month. This meant that you could get the coal in the winter without going out in the garden, a distinct improvement! The toilet was downstairs next to the 'coal hole'. There was no proper heating apart from the coal fire in the front room which heated the back boiler and hence hot water. No fire; no hot water!

My father, Harry, was a grocery manager at the local Blackley Co-operative Society. He earned 35 shillings a week, which was slightly above the average weekly wage at the time. He was also a local representative for USDAW (the grocers' Union of Shop Distributive and Allied Workers). Blackley Co-operative Society was variously known as the 'Stores'; the 'Co-op'; or the 'Coie'. The quarterly dividend they issued was an important supplement to the income of the working class inhabitants of

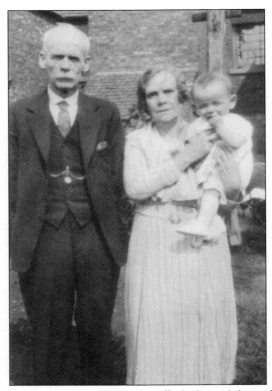

James Lee, my grandfather, the toffee boiler with his wife,
Elizabeth McGeckie, who holds me. Taken in mid-1935.

our area and was colloquially referred to as the Divi. My father would be upbraided in the street in later years when the Divi fell progressively from the dizzy heights of half a crown (12^{1}/$_{2}$p) in the pound to sixpence (2^{1}/$_{2}$p)!

Jean, my mother, stayed at home to look after us both. The only women in our area who went out to work were thought to be very low class, or 'common' and worked as cleaners, mill hands or at the cable or rubber works; all of these were very dirty occupations. Their husbands were thought not to be able (or willing) to provide for them. Allied to this condemnation of women who 'had' to go out to work, was a mistrust of any women who dressed, it was thought, too flashily. They were labelled in an equally pejorative manner as 'fur coats and no dinners' or 'fur coats and no knickers'!

I have two abiding memories of my fourth and fifth years (1938 and 1939). The first relates to the garden. My father came home one day from work and informed mother and me that an air raid shelter would be constructed in the back garden and the rest of the plot would be converted to growing potatoes for the Dig for Victory Campaign!

The arrival of the air raid shelter was a very big event in my young life. A lorry drew up loaded with corrugated iron girders, top soil and grass sods and within two days a magical den had been created fitted with a wooden door and wooden bunks. It was earthed over with sods and formed at first a natural hiding place and in later years a meeting point for the adolescent gangs which were an important part of my childhood. (See Chapter 4.)

After converting the garden to a large vegetable plot, my father decided that the windows of No. 24 needed protection against blast and he laboriously put lead strips inside all of them arranged in fancy geometric designs. Every house in the Avenue vied with each other to produce the best decorated windows! Whether these strips would have been any use at all in the event of a real blast is very doubtful.

My second abiding memory occurred in September 1939. I was on the beach at Ramsey in the Isle of Man outside my grandfather Jack's house (the Dogmills). Mother was on the beach too, no doubt keeping an eye on me and the Aberdeen terrier. My grandfather came down the garden by the little brook and out on to the beach. He said rather gruffly to my mother, 'Harry can't get over. They won't let him on the ferry'. It turned out later that this was the day after the outbreak of war and all British men of military age who were trying to get onto the ferries to the Isle of Man (or Ireland) were turned back at Liverpool. We left Ramsey hurriedly for the mainland and did not see my grandfather again for six years until the ferries were reopened for civilians in 1945. I heard later that my father then volunteered to join up (aged 34) but was rejected on two grounds: first his age, but then more particularly he was in a reserved occupation, that of a grocer.

My mother's change of countenance had reflected that something serious had happened but I did not fully realize the nature of this for another two years. War had been declared!

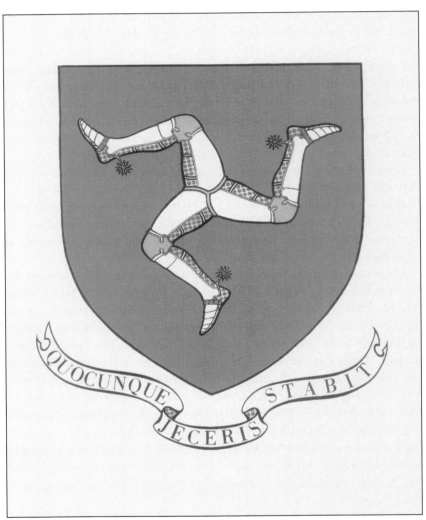

The Arms of the Isle of Man. 'Whithersoever you may have thrown it, it will stand.'

CHAPTER 2

The School, The War and Dad's Army

'Tis education forms the common mind. Just as the twig is bent
the tree's inclined.

Alexander Pope 1688-1744
Moral Essays Epistle 1.149

ON JANUARY 6th 1940 at the age of five years I enrolled at Victoria
Avenue Primary School, a large municipal barracks of a place with a
tarmac playground and an attached football field. Thus started a process of
formal education that was to last thirty years until I took the Doctor of
Philosophy and Doctor of Medicine degrees at Oxford University.

Initially I was in tears every morning for a fortnight but I gradually
settled down and made several friends who also lived in Tweedale Avenue.
Eventually we left our mothers behind and made the eight-hundred-yard
journey from home to school by ourselves forming small groups as we
went along. My initial separation anxiety was soon replaced by a sense of
excitement, which lasted throughout the whole war. First came the gas
mask drill. We were fitted with these contraptions by the teachers. I can
still remember the smell of rubber and the tight pressure that the mask
exerted on the sides of the head. At the sound of a handbell (or the air
raid warning from the siren on the local water tower) we had to don the
masks and get under the desks. If the raid was prolonged, we had to go
down to the basement and sit patiently on forms. At the sound of the 'All
Clear' the process was repeated in reverse. The school was also equipped
for blast and fire with sandbags, window taping, stirrup pumps and
strategically positioned heaps of sand. As we shall see later these measures
were of no benefit at all when the testing time came!

In spite of all these distractions education started and continued. There
were three impressively large men with large voices: Mr Cartledge, Mr
Liptrott and Mr Dunne (the headmaster). Discipline was enforced by
corporal punishment; Mr Cartledge and Mr Liptrott favoured a large

wooden ruler banged hard down on the knuckles; Mr Dunne administered the leather belt or strap. All administrations of the strap were entered in the Punishment Book (or PB), which developed a mythical significance of its own.

Tables were learned by rote with a peculiar chanting rhythm which rings in my ears to this day. Letters were copied out laboriously (fair copying) and sentences were repeated phonetically going round the illustrations that ran round the walls of the classrooms. Apart from an occasional story read aloud by the teacher and jumping round in a cold playground (so-called Physical Education) this was the sum total every day from nine in the morning to three thirty in the afternoon.

Fortunately I took to reading like the proverbial duck to water. There were very few books in our house apart from the Bible and a dictionary but my father took the *Daily Herald* in the morning and the *Manchester Evening News* at night. First with the headlines, then some of the sport, and progressively with the major battles (and disasters), I devoured the whole lot voraciously. This ignited a lifelong passion for newspapers which is with me to this day. If I am on holiday abroad I feel bereft if I cannot find a British paper. This led to the occasional funny incident. I can recall (at about the age of eight) reading something in the *Evening News* concerning prostitutes and asking my father what this word was all about! He passed it off, for me to discover the truth some years later.

This precocious ability to read resulted in my being taken to the local Public Library on Hill Lane. This I regarded as Aladdin's cave and the young female attendants as his acolytes. Starting off with Dr Dolittle, I proceeded over the course of time to Biggles and the Scarlet Pimpernel and then onto Captain Horatio Hornblower RN. This had two long term effects; first, I wanted to be a naval officer which, as we shall see, had to be rejected on the grounds of ill health, and secondly, I became a book lover. When I had, in later life, the money to indulge this love affair, I took up book collecting.

So far the war had had little impact on Blackley, though things were to change in 1941. I was puzzled about this lack of activity so I consulted my cousin Brian, who also lived in Tweedale Avenue and who at the age of eight or nine was the fount of all knowledge on matters concerning football, cricket, cigarette cards and the conduct of the war! He assured me that the Germans, led by the demon Adolph Hitler, would shortly be

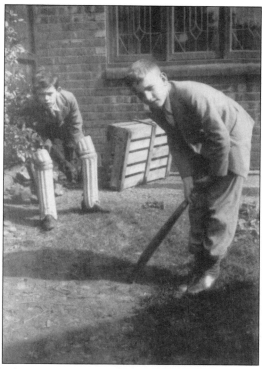

Cricket in the back garden at 24 in 1944. Brian Lee is at bat. The wicket keeper peers from behind an elderberry bush! Note the leaded lights on the windows (an antiblast device).

attacking and there would be fighting in the streets! This would be preceded by bombing attacks on Blackley and surrounding areas; in particular the Bowlee RAF camp and the AVRO works at Chadderton which manufactured airplanes. He had been told this with authority by his father Jim who was working as a crane driver and was a lynchpin in the war effort! Hitler had impinged on all of us boys as he was lampooned in the cartoons in the papers. We also sang with gusto, 'Hitler has only got one ball; whereas Goebbels has no balls at all!'

Brian's views were to prove inspired. In late 1941, just weeks later, the Luftwaffe began to attack Manchester. Night after night the air raid siren went and night after night we went into the shelter in the garden and stayed there till about four o'clock in the morning until the 'All clear' sounded. Much damage was done in central Manchester, and the docks and marshalling yards were hit. The nights were alive with the heavy thump of the bombers' engines and the crump-crump-crump of the anti-aircraft guns based in Heaton Park.

Brian and I thought this was great fun, being up all night. We had no fear and were too young to appreciate anxiety in our relatives. Supplies of broken biscuits were obtained from the biscuit factory and we munched away in a contented manner.

One night however Jerry got fairly close! In contrast to the faraway noise of attacks on Central Manchester, three high explosive bombs fell in and around our school demolishing several houses and killing three people. The school playground was also struck. As the bombs fell the whole air raid shelter shook with each impact and my father said, 'That was close!' In the morning we went off to school to find it closed with many windows blown out and a huge crater in the playground which had been roped off. A kindly ARP warden allowed us to peer into the hole, which seemed immense to a seven year old. A few weeks later there was a delayed result of the bombing. The school was evacuated to Blackpool and the Fylde Coast.

Brian and I did not go. Brian's parents did not want him to go with strangers and I was just recovered from rheumatic fever and my parents were understandably anxious about my health (see Chapter 3). The school returned in less than twelve months when it became clear that major night raids on provincial cities were over.

This absence of many of our school friends in Blackpool would have been thought to have resulted in boredom and frustration but in fact the exact opposite was the case. Two things helped to fill the next year. They were a bicycle and the Home Guard. A small bicycle enabled me to explore Blackley as far east as Heaton Park; as far west as the Avenue cinema, north to the mills of Rhodes and south to the anti-aircraft balloon in Lower Blackley. There was always something going on and later I was accompanied by my faithful Cairn Terrier Mac who was into everything, fought every dog he met and became my sibling and friend.

The next big excitement was the Home Guard. Father announced that he was joining the LDV which later became the Home Guard, and off he went to the Water Tower to do so. The next thing we knew he appeared in his khaki uniform and his cap with the badge of the 41st Company of the

Lancashire Fusiliers. The Company Commander was Captain Chapman (First World War veteran) and the Sergeant Major was Cliff Woods, ex Regimental Sergeant Major of the Coldstream Guards. At 6 ft 2 ins he was an imposing ramrod of a figure who rapidly became a close friend of my father. I used to go off and watch them drilling at the Water Tower site. I also imagined that Mac and I were semi-detached supporters looking for Nazi spies and the Fifth Column (whatever that was!).

Things got more exciting by the day: my father was issued with a 303 rifle and obtained his marksman's certificate. Then a Sten Gun appeared with 300 rounds of ammunition! This was stored in the hall of No. 24 and I was under a strict injunction not to play with it. Unsurprisingly I took no notice of this order at all and, when my parents were out, I used to race round the house with the empty Sten firing at German parachutists, hotly pursued by Mac who used to bark frantically.

There was much talk at the tea table about these German parachutists. The local top brass (i.e. Captain Chapman!) had been informed by the High Command that the enemy had targeted two local areas, Agecroft Power Station to disrupt the electricity supply and the reservoirs at Heaton Park in order to poison the water. Accordingly a guard would be mounted night and day at these strategic locations. Dad would do two nights a week as an armed guard at Heaton Park.

A couple of weeks later he came home in hoots of laughter. On the previous night whilst playing cards with Cliff Woods in the water bailiff's hut they were surprised to hear rifle fire. Cliff turned out the guard and they crept cautiously to where an eighteen-year-old private had been on watch. They found him shaking like a leaf, pointing his rifle away to a line of bushes close by the reservoir. He claimed that he had just shot an intruder who had failed to halt and failed to identify himself! Cliff Woods fanned out the platoon and they very cautiously crawled and scrambled down to where the mystery man was thought to be. Cliff Woods made the final assault, as befitted an ex-guardsman, and stumbled across a gardener's wheelbarrow! This was the German parachutist. The eighteen-year-old was sent off duty to recover his equanimity!

Increasingly the manoeuvres of the 41st Company had become more sophisticated. They blacked up their faces, imitated trees with green and brown camouflage and were issued with live ammunition. Brian and I on our bicycles followed them as best we could, getting told off occasionally when we were seen. However we knew the local area very well as we had played 'wide' games with the Cubs and reconnoitred every stream that flowed into the Irwell and every copse on the 'back fields' and in the parks.

In 1942 the Canadians arrived and in a large scale rehearsal attempted to take Agecroft Power Station. 41st Company together with other detachments of the local Home Guard defended this position. The action took place over forty eight hours from Saturday to Monday. Umpires decided who was dead, disabled or captured.

Needless to say the local Home Guard triumphed! The prairie boys simply did not know the terrain as well as the locals and got hemmed in down by the Irwell. The result gratified my father who took ten 'prisoners' personally. A few months later he was deeply affected when he discovered that many of these same young men had been killed when the Canadians sustained heavy losses at the landing at Dieppe on the French coast.

41st Company progressed steadily and became, to my young eyes, a fairly well disciplined outfit. It was decided by the 'High Ups' that they should have a band! Retired, decrepit and overweight brass bandsmen were summoned from Blackley, Moston, Failsworth and environs. They were stuffed with difficulty into their uniforms and started to rehearse with a motley collection of instruments at the meeting room at the Water Tower. Their marching was awful, but the playing rapidly improved under the aegis of a retired colliery bandmaster.

Once a month they paraded with 41st Company to St Paul's Anglican Church at the Avenue corner. This was marvellous! The strains of Colonel Bogey, Voice of the Guns and Lumberjack echoed over the route of the march. I was at the Water Tower waiting for them and would march down the pavement with them and then march back later on after the service was over. Initially, as always, Mac went with me but then he took a strong dislike to the big drum (and the big drummer) nipped out into the parade and bit him on the ankle. He was then banned and locked into 24 Tweedale, where he whined all morning.

I thought these military marches were magical and I liked particularly, 'Where are the Boys of the Old Brigade; where are the lads we fought with?' which was chosen by 41st Company as its special tune. Even today almost sixty years later if I hear this march I am transported to Victoria

Avenue and the Home Guard. After the war ended the band was kept going as the Home Guard Old Comrades and my father became President of the Association.

The war was progressing well. I knew this because once a fortnight, my parents and I used to take the 60 bus to Harpurhey to see Aunty Bertha and Uncle John. On the wall John had placed a large map of Europe and into it were stuck pins emblazoned with either the Swastika or the Union Jack. Throughout 1941, 1942 and 1943 our flags advanced across North Africa, into Sicily and up the spine of Italy.

Then came murmurs of a Second Front. The Allies were set to invade France or the Low Countries but nobody knew when and where. This gave rise to a rhyme that we lads used to repeat, 'I know a nursemaid down our street who knows a policeman on his beat who knows a man with a cat's meat cart who knows when the Second Front will start!' Eventually D-day came and I followed the results with breathless excitement. There were two main sources of information, the newsreels at the local Avenue Cinema, which we saw once or twice a week, and Uncle John's flags which advanced steadily across France from Normandy towards Paris.

All night-time air raids had been halted for over a year but in 1943 Hitler had made one last convulsive attack on Blackley! Within weeks of each other there were two daylight raids by fighter bombers aimed, once again, at Bowlee RAF Station and AVROs. In the second attack, the German plane flew directly over Tweedale Avenue, at rooftop level, presumably to get under the trajectory of the anti-aircraft fire. I was just returning to school after dinner but the plane was so low I could see the Nazi swastikas. Not much damage was done but this led to mobile anti-aircraft guns being deployed, which used to fire off from the backfields down by Longton Road shaking all the windows.

As we entered 1945 I was to suffer a bereavement. Mac, my five year old Cairn Terrier, was knocked down by a lorry on Victoria Avenue and killed. He had been under the nominal care of my cousin Dorothy, who returned from the scene in floods of tears. Mac had developed the stupid habit of attacking cyclists, cars and lorries. Normally cars and lorries were too quick for him but on this occasion the back wheels of the lorry had crushed him instantly spilling his guts on the road. Father took a sack from the 'coal hole', together with a spade and we went as a melancholy

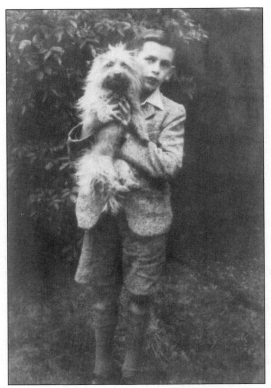

*The author, aged 11 years, with the second Cairn Terrier
'Sandy'. Note the bat ears and the Brylcreemed hair!*

procession to the Avenue, recovered the body and then went to the backfields to bury it. I was bereft. Mac had been to me, an only child, a brother and my constant companion in many adventures and escapades, including our counterespionage work! About nine months later the gap was filled by another Cairn Terrier, 'Sandy', who was in many ways just as mad as Mac.

In 1945 VE day came and a public holiday was declared. There was no widespread rejoicing in the city of Manchester although later, before being stood down, the Home Guard Units paraded with the local services before the Lord Mayor and associated worthies. In many ways my father was sorry when the Home Guard did come to an end. He had enjoyed it thoroughly and it was a welcome diversion from the boredom of rationing and the restrictions of the daily round he had to endure as a manager of a Co-operative store.

In the short term another diversion appeared to command his (and our) attention. Winston Churchill called the May 1945 General Election. My father, who at this time was an active Socialist, sprang into action and acted as a canvasser (and organizer) for Jack (John) Diamond the local Labour candidate. As boys, after a gang meeting, we decided also to support Labour and began a campaign of vandalism whose object was to get out in the twilight about eight o-clock at night and tear down all Conservative and Liberal posters. This sometimes involved altercations with their workers (and other gangs) but on our cycles we could be up and away very quickly! Jack Diamond was returned for Blackley with a comfortable majority and he suggested to my father that he should stand for Blackley as a local councillor when the next opportunity came around. As events will show, my father chose to withdraw from active politics when my mother became ill (see Chapter 3).

In June 1945 it was announced that the passenger ferries to the Isle of Man would reopen and in late July we set off for Douglas, via Fleetwood in North Lancashire. The train from Victoria Station was absolutely packed even though we had left at 6 o'clock in the morning to try and beat the rush. When we reached Fleetwood the station and the ferry terminal resembled a football crowd with people milling about in all directions. We were unable to get to the Island that day and had to book tickets for the day following. This meant an overnight stay in a bed and breakfast establishment near the old lighthouse. We tried to contact Grandad on the Island by telephone but without success!

The next day we sailed for the Island. The boat was packed and Brian my cousin was sick. Eventually we reached Douglas after about five hours to see Grandad on the quayside. It was the first time my mother (and I) had seen him for over 5 years since we left in September 1939. Visiting the Isle of Man was like going back in time. We travelled from Douglas to Ramsey on the electric tramway, a Victorian relic, with a top speed of about twenty miles an hour. We then had to walk with our suitcases about two miles up the Bride Road to Aunty Girlie's cottage where we were to stay. The cottage had no running water, and light was provided by paraffin oil lamps. In order to obtain water we had to go with a bucket to a spring in the field nearby, a distance of about one hundred yards. The toilet was

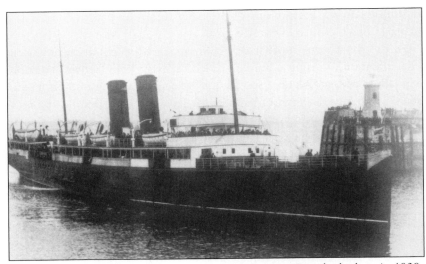

The Isle of Man Steam Packet Boat Mona's Isle *entering Douglas harbour in 1939.*

the night soil type in a shed in the back garden! Brian and I felt that we were living like pirates as the beach and the sea were only two hundred yards from the cottage. On going down there you could see the whole sweep of Ramsey Bay from the Maughold Head to the Point of Aire at the northern tip of the island. Grandfather's house, the Dogmills, was about half a mile further up the Bride Road. Here he lived like a retired sea captain with his sister Maggie, having long been a widower.

Billeted on him were two RAF sergeants from the nearby base at Andreas and this was the reason he had no room for us at the Dogmills. On one day they took Brian and me up to the observation post near the lighthouse, from which we watched the bombing runs on the practice area in the sea. They were in constant two-way communication with the base at Andreas and this to two young lads was high excitement indeed.

Grandad had a strict routine. In the morning he rose at 6 a.m., lit the fires, and chopped wood. At 8 a.m. he raised the Union Jack on his flagpole (now allowed again after VE day) and stood to attention for a moment as befitted a retired bosun in the Merchant Navy. Everyday he went twice into Ramsey with his two faithful dogs Metz and Jean, an Airedale and Aberdeen Terrier respectively. The trips to Ramsey involved shopping and ended in the local pub where he took two pints of mild ale.

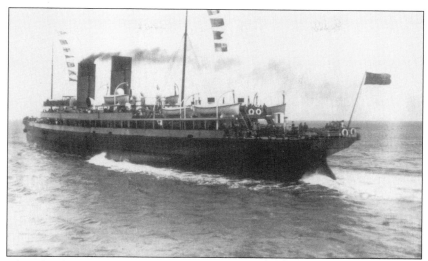

The Isle of Man Steam Packet Boat Viking *leaves for the mainland in August 1945 with flags flying to celebrate the end of the war.*

The same was repeated in the evening followed by flag lowering at 8 p.m., the BBC 9 o'clock news on the Home Service and so to bed. Occasionally he would drink whisky, or John Barleycorn, as he called it, and this might bring on a recitation of poetry by Burns. I will not forget the night he gave us the whole of Tam o' Shanter from memory!

Eventually the time came to return to Manchester and our piratical games were over. On reaching Douglas Harbour, all the fishing boats, tugboats and others were dressed overall with flags and bunting. As the ferry boat, the *Viking*, drew out for Fleetwood, all the assembled fleet, sounded their sirens in a blasting cacophony. It was VJ day! The war was over!

I had started the war on the beach in the Isle of Man and it had ended once again on the Island, this time at Douglas Harbour. I had no insight into the great loss of life, the Holocaust, the threat from Russia, displaced persons, or the evil Japanese empire. I simply regarded it as a 'jolly good show' and felt a sense of deflation as to what might happen next. One day I hoped to live in the Island again, this Nirvana of sea and hill, but it was not to be.

CHAPTER 3

Gangs, Injury and Illness

Is there no balm in Gilead;
is there no physician there?
Bible, Old Testament
Jeremiah 8.22

A N IMPORTANT PART of growing up in Tweedale Avenue was the 'gang'. This was a loose group of boys ranging from about nine to thirteen years who usually attended the same school and claimed a small geographical area of the estate as their fiefdom.

Our gang was based on Tweedale Avenue and Longton Road and its territory comprised these streets and part of the corporation 'tip' and the back fields. We were in conflict with the Crossfield gang and the Adiolas who abutted on our territory to the north and south respectively. The Adiolas had gained this sobriquet because of their rallying call Adi*ooo*la which they used to frightening effect!

Our gang consisted of two Brians, a Malcolm, a Robert, a Jack, a Clive, and myself, with occasional hangers on. The leader was Brian P. and his dominance was established by wrestling matches until the beaten individual was pinned to the ground and said 'Give in'. Most of our day-to-day activities involved building dens on the back fields, or 'swealing', and playing football and cricket. These activities must be described in more detail.

The den was the gang headquarters. We would burrow out a hole on the back fields, usually about six feet by four feet. This would be roofed with scrap timber and then the sides and roof completed with earthen sods. A well constructed den would last for months and the only real danger was marauding by other gangs who would tear the whole thing to pieces and steal the timber for their own constructions. The dens were very good hiding places where you could avoid parents, angry house-holders and, if necessary, the school attendance officer.

Swealing was setting fire to the grass and scrub on the back fields. This usually occurred in late August (or early September) and, if the grass was dry enough and there was some wind, resulted in a dramatic and satisfying blaze. Armed with matches, a small volume of methylated spirit and a few newspapers it was child's play to get a burn going. Often we would put the blaze out ourselves but occasionally it would get completely out of hand and the fire brigade had to be called. We were threatened with retribution by the authorities but as it was very difficult to identify the fire-setter and as there was no danger to life or property, nothing usually came of it.

Apart from this very entertaining activity most of our efforts were minor criminality, shooting out street lamps with catapults, pilfering from the local shop, Diamonds, and knocking on neighbourhood doors and running away.

One trick gave us great pleasure. We would tie a length of cotton to the knocker on the front door of the Hopwoods' house and stretch it out for about sixty feet and then hide behind the hedge on the opposite side of the road. Tweaking the knocker with the cotton and then letting it fall produced a satisfactory annoyance and puzzlement on Mr and Mrs Hopwoods' parts when they came to the door. Eventually Mr Hopwood complained to my father, who threatened me with a 'clip round the earhole' if I did not desist. On another occasion, aged about eleven, I was hiding in the back garden behind the defunct air raid shelter when my father who was planting sweet peas asked me, 'what the devil are you doing?'. I replied without a moment's hesitation that I was hiding from Mr Hopwood and that, 'discretion was the better part of valour'. I had no real idea what this meant but it sounded good. I wondered why my father fell about laughing!

Our gang had an unwritten code of conduct and behaviour. The first and most important rule was that we did not inform on or implicate other members of the gang – this was called being a 'tell-tale'. The second rule was that crying was a sign of weakness and was not to be tolerated. We staged impromptu boxing matches and 'tortured' each other in order to toughen up. The third rule was that we showed no enthusiasm for school work but great keenness for war, sport and feats of daring. The fourth rule was that certain activities were regarded as 'cissy' and were not to be tolerated. These cissy activities included anything to do with girls, dancing, piano lessons, singing apart from ribald scatological doggerel and even having a haircut. Terms of abuse were shouted at other gangs – they were 'mardy' (i.e. soft); cowardy-custards; sons of dogs (derived from pirate films); and had no spunk! The significance of this last insult escaped us.

The climax of the gang year was Bonfire Night (5 November). As soon as we returned to school in September, after the summer holidays were over, we began to collect cardboard boxes and scrap wood and to range over the back fields cutting down branches of trees. All this material was brought from many points of the compass to the site on Longton Road where there was an area of waste ground, next to the entrance to the corporation tip. Slowly the edifice would rise until by the end of October it reached 20 to 30 feet.

In October gang activity became frenzied. One group would be away collecting materials, one group would be outside Diamonds collecting a penny for the Guy and the last and most important group would be guarding the bonfire.

The rival gangs looked upon each other's bonfires with envious eyes. Waiting till near dusk there were two manoeuvres. The first would be to steal material from another bonfire and the second, equally effective, would be to damage the bonfire by setting fire to it prematurely.

In the last week the adults who lived in Longton Road entered into the struggle as well! Mrs Johnston whose kitchen window overlooked the waste ground where the bonfire was situated would drive off suspicious youths or boys. A collection was also taken from the neighbours to finance the purchase of fireworks, sweets and chestnuts. The ladies of the locale would make treacle toffee and bake the North Country heavy cake parkin.

In the weeks before the 5th we would purchase 'bangers' and 'ripraps'. These were used as offensive weapons. The technique was as follows – on meeting rival gangs you would light a banger in the right hand, wait till the fuse spluttered and then throw it towards the 'enemy'. If timed properly this would create a very satisfactory bang. The 'rip-rap' was similar but on igniting would jump about like a flailing dervish. Occasionally rockets would be launched horizontally from milk bottles to fire into the bonfires of the opposition. Obviously these practices were very dangerous and bangers and rip-raps are now banned. Eventually the great night would come and we would sing 'Remember Remember the 5th of November; Gunpowder Treason and Plot! Can you give Good Reason why Gunpowder and Treason should ever be forgot'. The bonfire would be lit in several places with the judicious application of methylated spirits (if the weather had been wet). The flames leapt many feet into the air and the fireworks flared. Parkin, toffee and chestnuts were consumed. The adults supervised the safe burning of the bonfire and the police and fire brigade turned a blind eye to proceedings, provided that there was no obstruction to Longton Road. The bonfire would still be burning next morning with the ashes glowing white hot. We would stand round it with some feeling of 'let down'. It was all over for another year!

On one Bonfire night the Lee family almost sustained a casualty. Our second Cairn Terrier Sandy escaped from the house, although how he did it remains a mystery. His latent aggression stimulated by the banging, he headed straight for the crowd. Next minute, I heard a yelp and saw that Mr Lomas a near neighbour had kicked him in the ribs! It transpired later that Sandy seeking somebody (or something) to fight with had picked up a riprap in his mouth. Mr Lomas, thinking very quickly, had kicked Sandy in the ribs just before the firework exploded and the offending object had come out of the dog's mouth like a cork out of a bottle. Sandy would have had his jaw blown off or, at the very least, sustained serious injuries to his mouth. As it was, the dog survived until he was fourteen years of age and died peacefully in his box.

I was to be one of the casualties of gang warfare. Normally, as I have said, gang rivalry consisted of hurling insults or throwing fireworks at each other. Occasionally it turned nasty and involved stone throwing. One line of dispute was where the corporation tip met the stream and the land rose towards the estate where the Crossfielders lived.

On this particular day, we lined up at the top of the tip and the opposition, the Crossfielders, on their rising ground beyond the stream. Insults led to stone throwing and by a fluke, a slate hit me above the right eye and my face was pouring with blood. I was hauled off home and our gang, enraged, went and captured the miscreant who had launched the missile and he was forced to come to 24 Tweedale to apologize.

Mother bandaged the wound as best as she was able but when my father came home from work he took one look at it, picked me up on his shoulders and carried me down to the local surgery to see Dr Howitt our general practitioner. He also gave it a cursory inspection and sent me straight to the Manchester Eye Hospital by taxi. I had nine stitches in the eyebrow and the Resident Surgical Officer pronounced himself satisfied that there was no internal damage to the eye. However this goes to show how wrong doctors can be! As I shall describe later, this eye was to prove a continuing problem up to the present day.

The next setback in health was to be more pressing than a few stitches (and a night at the Eye Hospital). It was rheumatic fever, also known as acute rheumatism. The first episode occurred when I was four years old and I have no memory of it at all. The second episode at the age of seven years had an indelible effect on both my life and my choice of career. I used to get regular sore throats but on this particular occasion, about a week after the bout of painful swallowing, I woke up with a painful right knee and two days later I had pain (and swelling) in the left ankle. I was to learn later that this is the characteristic 'flitting' arthritis of rheumatic fever. I also felt slightly out of sorts and my mother informed me, after wielding the mercury thermometer, that my temperature was 100°F. Dr Howitt, our general practitioner, was summoned and he arrived in a large overcoat (and Homburg) to be treated with great deference by my mother.

He examined my joints; looked at my throat; listened to my heart carefully and then pronounced with grave certainty, 'Your son has rheumatic fever. He should go to hospital'. My mother resisted this prospect of separation and, reluctantly, Dr Howitt agreed that I could be nursed at home. This would however involve the following: my bed to be brought downstairs; an enforced twelve-week rest; to get up only to go to the commode; and, if any deterioration occurred, I was to go straight to hospital.

This was a very impressive performance on the doctor's part (like a fiat or imprimatur) and I was bowled over, particularly as I did not feel really ill. The next development was the arrival of the 'medicine' from the local chemist. This proved to be the most bitter substance I had ever taken in my life with a very pronounced after-taste. I usually persuaded my mother to give me a 'sweet' to take away the awful effects and the reflex salivation. In retrospect it was probably sodium salicylate, the bitter principle from the bark of the willow Salix.

At first being confined to bed was very pleasant and appealed to my

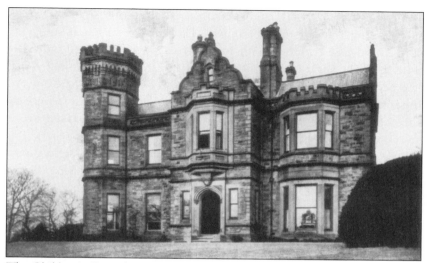

The Children's Convalescent Home in Cheshire. Here I spent a miserable period early in 1942.

innate laziness. Sandy, my Cairn Terrier, joined me in and on the bed and we played games of 'find the rat' which involved him burrowing into the bed clothes. There was also time for reading three books a week from the Public Library and my word power improved considerably.

Towards the end of the second month I began to get bored, but the regime could not be relaxed. Dr Howitt informed my mother that my heart was damaged and that I had a 'cardiac murmur'. This had several consequences: that I should not undertake any physical activity of a strenuous nature such as swimming and football. For the first six months I should pause halfway up our twelve stairs, and that for a year I should walk up all hills backwards!

Eventually I was released from the prison of bed but the prolonged inactivity had made my leg muscles very weak and I had developed fallen plantar arches. The first step the School Medical Officer said was that I must go 'convalescent'. Manchester Education Authority had a convalescent home in Bollington some fifteen miles south of the city. Two weeks was the sentence! The day came when I had to go to Cheshire and leave mother, home, and Sandy. We trooped off to London Road Railway Station and I remember the deep sense of sadness I felt.

The home was run on regimental lines and most of the children were older, stronger and potential dangers. The meals were communal and awful; hard-faced women with loud voices served porridge with salt rather than the sugar to which I had been accustomed. I was singled out by everybody, staff and convalescents, because I could not take part in any games (or activities) demanding physical activity, and also because I had to walk up hills backwards on the country walks that were taken every afternoon as 'constitutionals'!

I was glad to return to Blackley and my parents. The next episode was to attend remedial orthopaedic classes for my fallen arches. These included walking on the beam, swinging on ropes and vaulting over low horses. The orthopaedic assistants paid no attention to the embargo on my physical activity and sixty years later, as I look back, I doubt very much whether twelve weeks in bed, walking up hills backwards, or spending a fortnight in rural Cheshire made one iota of difference to the eventual outcome! I had simply been lucky that the inflammation on the mitral valve in the left side of the heart had not progressed to significant narrowing (a potentially serious complication called mitral stenosis).

There were some benefits from the diagnosis of my 'damaged' heart. As an only child I was always spoiled by my parents, in particular by my mother, but after my eye injury and then the rheumatic fever I was overprotected and everything was done for me. This has made me incurably lazy and also self-centred. I shall discuss these character deficiencies later in this memoir.

Another illness was to play an important part in my life as I started grammar school at the age of almost twelve years. My mother, who normally had a sunny and equable temperament, began to change in personality. She became progressively grumpy and bad tempered. Then the housework began to suffer; she could no longer do the heavy washing on Mondays with the copper boiler; shortness of breath ensued and eventually some ankle swelling. There were blazing rows with my father, during which my mother accused him of treating her as a 'skivvy'. A painful corneal ulcer developed which was slow to heal.

Dr Howitt was asked to visit after a few months of gradual deterioration. He confessed himself puzzled but asked his assistant, Dr Jelenowicz, a displaced Polish doctor, to review my mother's problems. He had been an ophthalmologist in his native Poland and he examined my mother's

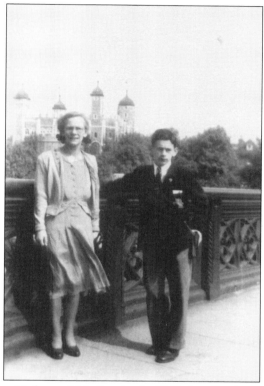

*Mother and I in London in 1947. Jean Lee has
undiagnosed pernicious anaemia and looks awful!*

eyes with an ophthalmoscope which I found fascinating. He then said in broken English, 'You will require a blood test'.

We take such things for granted nowadays but in 1948 this involved a journey to the Northern Hospital some three miles away, and as such was a major undertaking. A week later the result came back; my mother was grossly anaemic. Dr Sam Oleesky, a 'specialist', admitted her to the Jewish Hospital in nearby Salford where she had several blood transfusions and a bone marrow test.

My father returned from the hospital one evening to announce that mother had pernicious anaemia and this would involve lifelong injections of concentrated liver extract. This diagnosis of 'pernicious' anaemia both baffled and intrigued me. I looked up pernicious in the dictionary to find

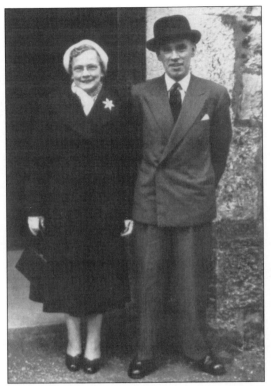

*My parents in better times (1960). Mother has put on weight. Father favours
the headgear popular at that time with Cooperative Society managers!*

it defined as destructive, highly injurious or malevolent, derived from the
Latin pernicious – death by violence. Anyway mother responded
dramatically, both physically and mentally, to the liver injections. She
gained two stones in weight; her hair darkened and her sunny personality
reappeared. Later, concentrated liver was replaced by pure vitamin B_{12}
which my mother had regularly every two months, until she died from
other causes in 1975 some thirty years later.

These illnesses had a great impact on me and raised all sorts of
questions. What was rheumatic fever and how did it damage the heart?
Why was pernicious anaemia so dangerous? How did concentrated liver
'cure' the condition? What was this marvellous substance with the
beautiful red colour called vitamin B_{12}? Nobody in our family understood

it. Even Aunty Amy who was matron of the Eye Hospital at Nottingham could not give explanations that satisfied a twelve-year-old. I resolved for a second time that I would become a doctor and then I would understand everything!

I consulted both my father and my Uncle Eric, who had returned from the Forces to train as a teacher. How did you become a doctor? The answer came back clearly, you must go to the University and study medicine. I had no real insight into what these simple statements implied but I resolved that if this is what had to be done, then it would be done!

CHAPTER 4

Methodists, Proddydogs and Catolicks

Only an armour bearer firmly I stand,
Ready to follow at the King's command
If in the battle to my trust I am true
Mine shall be the Honours in the Grand Review
Old Methodist hymn

IN ORDER TO DILUTE the influence of the gang (and gang loyalty) my
parents decided that they must try and infiltrate my beliefs with aspects
of Christian doctrine.

Mother had been confirmed in the Church of England in Bootle,
Liverpool and sporadically attended St Paul's Anglican Church on the
Avenue corner. Father had been brought up as a Methodist in Lower
Crumpsall, Manchester. It was decided on nondoctrinal grounds that I
should go to Hopkinson Road Independent Methodist Chapel Sunday
School, simply because it was only 400 yards from Tweedale. I accepted
this decision with some reluctance as it would interfere with my activities
on a Sunday. Several other members of the gang were dragooned in a
similar way.

Hopkinson Road Chapel was an interesting institution. It consisted of a
large assembly hall with several small rooms off it. There was no altar or
communion rail but a small central table and a pulpit but no dais. There
was one simple cross on the wall but no other decoration. Music was
provided by a harmonium.

The lynchpin of the Chapel was the Abbott family. They lived in
Tweedale and three times a day on Sundays they would be up at
Hopkinson Road holding services. They cleaned, raised money and
evangelized. My father, who was a beer drinking Methodist and spent his
Sunday lunchtimes in the Lion and Lamb public house, admired them
greatly. The services were extremely simple: three or four hymns, usually
of a rousing nature; a few extempore prayers; a lesson from the Old and

26

New Testaments; and a fiery fifteen minute sermon. There were no creeds and I cannot remember any sacraments apart from the occasional baptism.

Our God was definitely Old Testament and there was a concentration on sin and the Ten Commandments. Drinking alcohol was a grievous sin and the body should be kept as pure as a sacred tabernacle. Later on I understood this was a vague reference to abstinence from masturbation although the word and the practice was never described in detail!

I enjoyed the lusty singing and the occasional debate we had about faith and works. I remember asking one of the Abbott brothers if somebody obeyed all the Commandments, prayed to God daily and observed the Golden rule but never set foot in Church would they go to Heaven? He paused for a moment (or two) and then replied that he (or she) would definitely be admitted. When I got home, I announced to my parents that this is what I proposed to do, but they were unconvinced! It is doubtful if our allegiance to Hopkinson Road would have been maintained for too long, if it had not been for some very positive features. These were the Sunday School outings, the Christmas parties and the 199th Scout troop.

The Sunday School trips and the Christmas parties were the highlights of the Hopkinson Road calendar. Twice a year the Abbott brothers would subsidize outings. In the winter this would be to the pantomime (or Belle Vue circus) and in the summer to Heaton Park or Ashworth Valley. Ashworth Valley was the favourite and most exciting destination. A Lancashire clough, with deep sides which were well wooded, it lent itself to all sorts of games and it was possible to paddle and build dams in the brook at the bottom.

A more long lasting influence was the 199th Cub and Scout troop which met in a hut by the side of the Chapel. I was banned from hard physical games like British Bulldog, skittle ball and tag games but I used to watch with interest.

A brass band was formed and this improved when two very old Scouts were drafted in, Kenderdine on top cornet and Jackman on trombone. Malcolm, Clive and Brian J took up the cornet. I had wished to do so but as a result of having no 'lip' and my previous rheumatic fever, I could not manage it. This was my first major disappointment but I travelled as a 'hanger on' when the band played in the Whit Week walks and elsewhere.

There were two major bonding occasions in the calendar year; Remembrance Sunday and Whitsun. In the years immediately following the war several hundred people would parade to the local war memorial led by the Old Comrades band (Harry Lee President!). In the middle would come the 199th Scout band and bringing up the rear would be the St Paul's Anglican Boys Brigade Band. This last was regarded as very much inferior as they only had bugles and drums!

The main parades in Manchester were those associated with Whitsuntide and colloquially known as the 'Walks'. On Whit Sunday the Anglicans in Blackley walked in witness; on Monday the Anglicans in the City; on Friday the Roman Catholics in the City; on Trinity Sunday Holy Trinity Moston (known irreverently to us as the Holy Tripe Shop); and various others at different times. The warehouses, offices and factories in Manchester routinely took a week's holiday at this time and much preparation went into girls' dresses, women's outfits, floral decorations and banners. It was an equivalent to the Wakes Week in the Lancashire cotton towns but with the important difference that the population did not migrate to the seaside at Blackpool but stayed in and around the city.

Apart from the great holiday atmosphere for the whole of Whit Week there were two other important aspects. First, it allowed adolescent boys to meet prepubertal (and pubertal) girls and second it underlined the rivalry between Protestant and Catholics, as to who could stage the most impressive parade.

Blackley (and Manchester in general) had a large immigrant Irish Catholic population. They lived mostly in the inner city areas of Ancoats, Collyhurst, Ardwick, Harpurhey and Hulme. Many of them had come over after the Great Potato Famine of the 1840s to find work in the mills and factories. In the 1870s the Fenians had shot a policeman dead in the city and this was referred to as an 'atrocity' by the Protestants. Several Fenians had been hanged and these were referred to as the Manchester Martyrs by the Roman Catholics. Every year there was a pilgrimage to the Martyr's memorial in a local cemetery. Following the Easter Rising in 1916 there had been some rioting in the city, particularly when the Mayor of Cork died after a hunger strike.

In the 1940s tension still ran high. The failure of De Valera (and Ireland) to enter the war against the Nazis, the flight of some Irishmen (and women) back to Eire, and the trouble over the Irish ports, all fuelled

Protestant distrust and hatred for the Irish Catholics. These grievances, coupled with the fact that the Pope was an Italian (and he had not condemned Mussolini) all served to transfer our attitudes (derived from those of our parents) to the local Catholic boys. In Blackley primary education was strictly segregated. At the top of Plant Hill, a few hundred yards from Tweedale Avenue, was St Claire's Roman Catholic Primary School which was run by the Franciscan friars.

Our gang passed the Catholic boys as they made their way to St Claire's and we made ours to the Avenue School. Normally there was some name-calling; we would shout Catolicks, potato pickers or bogtrotters, whereas they would shout Proddydogs, squareheads or bloody heathen! This was as far as hostilities went normally, with the insults hurled across the main road. Occasionally in the winter there would be snowballs and on one occasion the aggression erupted into a major battle with stone throwing and fist fighting. This last episode prompted Mr Dunne the headmaster to call the ten and eleven-year-olds to a special meeting where he threatened us with retribution unless we mended our ways. We readily acquiesced in this but had no intention of ceding any territory to the Catolicks in the long run!! Segregation would continue at the secondary level after the Eleven Plus examination. The Catholic boys went to St Bede's College or Xaverian, Protestant boys to North Manchester High School or Domett Street, and never the twain would meet except occasionally on the soccer or rugby football fields.

Our next-door neighbours were Roman Catholics and my father, while maintaining a polite exterior, was rabidly anti-Catholic. Privately he called them papists, Barks and Tagues and was full of all sorts of prejudices. They were trying to take over by outbreeding us (no contraception); they were priest-ridden; they behaved badly by heavy drinking and gambling and were able to have these sins too readily forgiven at confession; all Protestants were condemned by their church to perdition (*ex ecclesia nulla salus*); the Pope was Anti-Christ, and so on.

He particularly condemned the practice of mixed marriages and the harsh Romish regulations in regard to this. He had several employees who had 'turned' in order to marry a Catholic girl and, failing that, some who had agreed to have any children they might have brought up in the Faith of our Fathers.

Mother was less rabid but she had been brought up in Liverpool where tensions were high across the sectarian divide. Several of her relatives belonged to the Orange lodge and marched with triumphalist gusto, on 12 July, to commemorate the battle of the Boyne Water. My father was also somewhat paranoid about the Catholics in the Co-op and in the Labour Party. He had, after the war, been elected to the management board at the Co-op and was also an official USDAW representative. He thought a particular Catholic family were trying to infiltrate both the union and party organizations and this exercised him greatly! I thought all these opinions and reactions perfectly normal and it was ironic that, later on, when I fell in love with a Catholic girl, they would give me great trouble and anguish.

Some thirty years later, after my mother died, in the 1970s, my father, who was alone and lonely, still living in Blackley, was befriended by a Catholic couple and he came to value both their faith and support. In short he became convinced of the value of ecumenism! As for myself, who later became a republican agnostic, I now consider how stupid it all was and how divisive the sectarian schools were. Nobody goes to church now in Blackley and the present problems in South Lancashire have shifted to the ancient enmity between Muslim and Christian.

CHAPTER 5

Sporting Moments:
The Reds, the Blues and the Roses

And I look through my tears
on a soundless – clapping host
As the run stealers flicker to and fro
To and fro:- O my Hornby
and my Barlow long ago!
                    Francis Thompson 1859-1907
                                At Lord's

FROM THE END of the war to about 1950, the activities of our Gang were totally dominated by street sports, in rank order: football, then cricket, and then boxing.

Longton Road was our chosen arena as it was flatter and straighter than Tweedale and also because it provided an escape route to hide from angry neighbours in our 'den' or in the sandpits. The other advantage was there was very little through traffic apart from coal and grocery deliveries. The main obstacle to our efforts were the two policemen who lived in Longton, Inspector Collinge who was very severe on us and Constable Parker who was ambivalent. Luke Parker was regarded by us with awe as he was a giant of a man; 6 ft 3 ins tall and 17 stone. He was the anchor man in the police tug of war team; could pick up a constable under either arm and when he lifted an average cricket bat it seemed to be about the size of a rolling pin. He encouraged us to play cricket on the back fields but we refused to do this as the 'bounce' was so uneven that a good length ball could become either a bouncer or a 'grubber' (our term for a shooter).

Football dominated eight months of the year; cricket the remaining four. We would have played from dawn to dusk if we could but the exigencies of school prevented this. Soccer had two main variants, picking sides and an unusual game called 'one ball kick'.

31

Picking sides started with two captains having alternate choices after spinning a coin as to who would start. It did not matter if there were uneven numbers like five versus four, or six versus five. One boy, who was overweight and clumsy, was always chosen last with the statement, 'I suppose I'll have to take S'. I was usually chosen somewhere in the middle, neither good nor bad, but I had a slight advantage in that I was naturally a 'leftie' (left-footed), whereas everybody else was right-footed.

We usually played with a tennis ball and the goals were kept by Adge and Brian J who fancied themselves as natural custodians. The ball flew all over the place on the hard concrete and it was amazing that no one was seriously injured apart from a few bruises and damaged shins. There was no kit, no shin guards and no offside. Fouls were decided by general consensus as there was no referee. This led to a lot of shouting but there was surprisingly an inherent sense of fair play.

One ball kick was played when only two or three could gather together. It was a head-to-head contest and you were allowed only one kick at the ball and your opponent tried to block the shot with feet or body. The strike would then revert to your opponent. This game involved a lot of skill in playing off fences and walls or trying to flick the ball over your opponent's head. Usually we played first person to get three goals would win but this could easily take half an hour. Abuse of the players was common, either by an opponent or by interested spectators. This is when I first became aware that I had protuberant ears as I was heckled with, 'Jug Ears', 'Dumbo' or 'like a taxi with the doors wide open'. I in turn would should insults like, 'Fatty Arbuckle', 'Specky Four-Eyes' or 'Slowcoach'.

In May the cricket gear would come out. I say gear but this is a gross exaggeration! It consisted of a couple of battered cricket bats and an old box for a wicket. There were no pads or batting gloves – these did not materialize until we arrived at Secondary School. Our knowledge of the Rules was fragmentary and there were endless disputes about LBW!

Nevertheless we enjoyed it immensely and played every night until it was almost pitch dark. We were always aware of the threat of angry neighbours and the advent of Inspector Collinge or Constable Parker. On one occasion I received a rising ball on leg stump and hooked it straight through square leg and onto the Braithwaite's front window. The thud reverberated up and down Longton Road. Fortunately the window did not break as it was a tennis ball. We vamoosed at record speed and hid in the back fields while Mr Braithwaite tried to locate us. He never had a chance! Needless to say play was suspended for the day.

Our growing interest in sport was reflected by the resumption of professional activities in the city. Manchester had two great football teams, the United and the City. The United played in red shirts and white shorts (hence the Reds) and City in sky blue shirts and white shorts (hence the Blues). Before the war the Blues had had the better of things, winning the FA Cup in 1934. My father, who was a Blues supporter, talked lovingly of Swift in goal, Matt Busby at half-back and Alex Herd the centre forward.

The talk now was all about whether City would continue their dominance as football resumed in season 1945-1946. United were in a sorry state as their ground Old Trafford had been badly bomb damaged. City generously offered their ground, Maine Road, as a temporary home and for several seasons both clubs played their home games there until Old Trafford was repaired. United appointed a new manager, Matt Busby, who had previously been a City player. How would be do?

My first memory of football is my cousin Brian taking me to Maine Road early in 1946. It was a great adventure. First the 60 bus down into the city and then we had to get a tram from Piccadilly to the match. As we neared the terminus, Brian spotted a moving tram with its destination board labelled 'Maine Road' and said 'run for it'. Grabbing the central pole he went on to the running board first and I followed, being hauled aboard by him. This was known as 'decking on', a dangerous practice! When we arrived at Maine Road my memories are fragmentary. I remember very little about the match itself but several things made a deep impression. The first was the scores of trams lined up to take the spectators away; the second was the turnstiles and how hard they were to push; and the third was the shouting of the crowd in unison, 'Two; four; six; eight; who do we appreciate? U-N-I-T-E-D!' I was immediately a fan and, almost sixty years later, I still am.

Busby began to build a team, as servicemen returned from Europe and the Far East. Jimmy Delaney on the right wing came from Glasgow Celtic, Gentleman Johnny Carey came from the fair city of Dublin and Jack Rowley came from the South. Eventually the team settled down as follows: Crompton; Carey and Aston; Cockburn; Chilton, Anderson; Delaney, Morris, Rowley, Pearson and Mitten. They were all heroes to us but my particular favourite was Charlie Mitten on the left wing as this

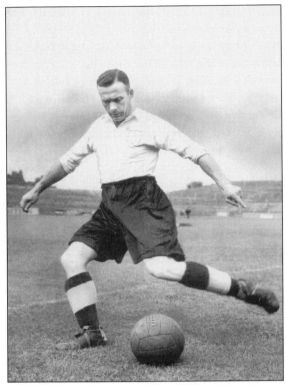

Charlie Mitten of Manchester United; Bogota and Fulham.
Also known as the 'Penalty King' and the 'Bogota Bandit'.

was the position I began to play at Secondary School. He was fast and elusive, could cross beautifully or alternatively cut inside and shoot. A modern equivalent would be Ryan Giggs also of Manchester United.

In season 1947/48 came the first real post-war success when United progressed steadily through the rounds of the FA Cup and reached a crucial game against Preston North End. Tom Finney, the Preston plumber, was the lynchpin of the North Lancashire side. Good with both feet, many informed observers thought he was a better player than the famous Stanley Matthews.

Brian obtained two tickets for the match. How I do not know as they were like gold dust. We turned up early and there was hardly anybody in the ground but as the time moved round to the 3 p.m. kick off, 75,000 people crammed into the stadium. I never have been so scared in my life! I could not see and I could not move. Aged thirteen, I was totally hemmed in. When the crowd surged forwards and back as an attack came on the goal below us, if anyone had gone down there would have been a tragedy.

Even getting out of the ground was an ordeal. The crowds funnelled through narrow gates and if you were in the centre you were simply carried along with no control of what happened. When I reached home, I was sick with anxiety and it took me a couple of days to recover. My parents realized that I had been crushed and, ever afterwards, I have disliked large crowds. The lessons at football grounds were of course disregarded for years – one only has to quote the deaths at Bolton, Ibrox Glasgow and Hillsborough Sheffield. United had won the cup tie against Preston by a narrow margin but that did not seem important at the time.

Eventually, after a few weeks, I recovered and by that time United had progressed to the Final of the Cup, where they were to play Blackpool, who in many ways were the favourites as they had in their team the great Stanley Matthews and a fine centre forward called Mortensen. For the whole week before the match I was in a ferment of anxiety until finally the day of reckoning came on the Saturday. Father and I settled down to listen to the match on the radio but when United fell behind, two goals to one, I simply could not bear the anxiety and the excitement any longer and I had to go out in the garden, where I lay down between the vegetables and contemplated the bursting of my dream. A few minutes later father came to the back door and shouted, 'United have equalized'. I still could not bring myself to go inside but when another shouted message came from the door that the Reds had gone ahead, I went indoors. Finally we won, four goals to two. The Cup was ours!

The following day several of the gang went down to Albert Square in the city centre, with many thousands of others, to see the Cup brought back to the Town Hall, and on the Wednesday the Avenue Cinema was packed to relive the highs and lows via the medium of the Pathe Newsreel. As the winning goals went in on the screen the whole audience stood and cheered.

We followed this United Team onto 1952-53, when they won the League Championship, and we invaded the pitch at Old Trafford. I then gradually lost interest in attending live matches, although I was at

Wembley in 1958 when United lost to Bolton Wanderers with the scratch team they had to put out after the Munich disaster. Even to this day, around 5 o'clock on a Saturday, I still look or listen out for Manchester United's result.

In the summer of 1946, thoughts turned to cricket and we began to go to Lancashire's ground at Old Trafford on a regular basis. Armed with sandwiches and a bottle of 'pop' we would make our way to the ground via the electric railway that stopped at Warwick Road Station. From there it was only a stone's throw to get into the ground – indeed Learie Constantine had once hit a ball out of the field and into the railway station. Lancashire was building up its team once again after the war, in an attempt to displace the old enemy, Yorkshire from the proud position of invincibility that it had held throughout the 1930s.

Our particular favourites were Cyril Washbrook and Winston Place, the Lancashire opening batsmen. On one occasion they made 350 for the first wicket, a Lancashire record, and we followed every run of it over the course of two days. Washbrook was the more flamboyant of the two batsmen with his hooking and pulling, whereas Place was better on a tricky wicket with his long reach and good defence. We were delighted when Washbrook was picked to join the record-breaking Len Hutton (Yorkshire) to open the England batting. Things were going very well but we had not bargained for Bradman's Australians in 1948.

As a result of the war the Aussies had not been to England since 1938 and their visit was eagerly anticipated. England's undoing was the opposition's deadly fast bowling duo Ray Lindwall and Keith Miller, together with the great catching by Don Tallon, the wicket-keeper and the slip fieldsmen. On the day of the Old Trafford Test Match, we got up at 6 a.m. and set off for the ground. The crowds were immense and had to be controlled by mounted policemen but we finally made it through a turnstile. Inside the ground the crowd was equally vast and we had to sit between a rope and the perimeter fence. If any ball was hit in the air, the whole crowd would rise and a great gasp would go up until it was either caught, dropped, or went over the boundary. Dennis Compton was fielding within ten yards of us and he complained that his new cricket boots were hurting him!

Australia batted first. Barnes collapsed at the wicket and had to retire hurt. Bradman made a modest score but Arthur Morris held the

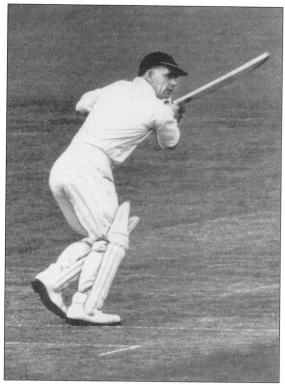

Cyril Washbrook of Lancashire and England.
A characteristic shot through the offside.

Australians together. England were in with a chance for the first time in the series.

Washbrook and Jack Crapp opened for England. Crapp was soon out to a 'snorter' from Lindwall. A cathedral-like hush descended on the ground as the great fast bowler ran in and when the ball was delivered there would be a great roar whatever happened to the delivery. It was like a fight between gladiators at the Roman Colosseum. Bradman had put Hassett back to deep fine leg and, knowing Washbrook's penchant for hooking, instructed Lindwall to fire in an occasional leg stump bouncer. Down came the bouncer! Washbrook hooked uppishly to Hassett who, accompanied by a mighty roar from the crowd, dropped the catch. Two overs later, the same ploy was repeated. Down came the bouncer!

Washbrook duly hooked for the second time and Hassett, receiving the catch at midriff height, promptly dropped the ball again! Hassett asked a policeman if he could borrow his helmet to catch the ball and Bradman the captain, fielding at mid-off, looked as though he had swallowed a frog.

England gained an advantage on the second day but the match was washed out with rain. Australia took the series four to nil (much to our disgust). My cricket watching continued till 1950 when Lancashire had a half share (with Surrey) in the County Championship.

Other matters began to take over and football and cricket faded away. My right eye was lazy after the injury and had a latent squint and my left eye slowly developed significant myopia. I was advised to wear glasses but out of vanity refused to do so. This refusal was to handicap me significantly, as I could not see the cricket ball. My lack of depth perception due to the severe imbalance between the two eyes was later to prove a destructive handicap in practical procedures such as dissection and surgical procedures.

I came to realize, reluctantly, that I would not be a Charlie Mitten or a Cyril Washbrook and that I must seek a middle-class education. I returned to my first love. By hook or by crook I would become a doctor. Where should I start?

CHAPTER 6

Education, Education and Education

'Reeling and Writhing to begin with' the Mock Turtle replied 'and
then the different branches of Arithmetic – Ambition, Distraction,
Uglification and Derision'.

Lewis Carroll 1832-1898
Alice In Wonderland
Chapter 9

RICHARD COBDEN, the Manchester radical, wrote to Tait in 1837 that
'education, education, education is the motto of every enlightened
democrat' and at his school, near his manufactory in Sabden, around the
walls were slogans announcing that 'education is the birthright of man'.

My father had passed the scholarship in the 1920s but his father, a
toffee boiler at the CWS works in Lower Crumpsall, could not afford to
send him to the Grammar School. As a consequence he left school at
fourteen years and joined Blackley Co-operative Society as a sugar boy,
weighing out two-pound bags of this commodity all day long. He claimed
his record was 375! From there over many years he eventually worked
himself up to be grocery manager at CRS (Blackley).

He vowed constantly that he never wanted to see me behind a grocer's
counter and that I should pass the scholarship and go to Owens College.
To dyed-in-the-wool Mancunians, Owens College was the preferred
name for what had become the Victoria University of Manchester. His
clearly expressed hope was that I should become an accountant as he had
met these professionals in business.

The big test was now to come. Early in 1946, at the age of eleven years
and three months (i.e. 11 plus) I took the examination at the Avenue
School with all my class companions – which would separate the sheep
from the goats. Of this examination I have no memories but I certainly
recall the other two examinations that I took at about the same time; the
entrance Scholarships to Manchester Grammar School and to William

Hulme's Grammar School. These latter two schools were the premier boys' schools in Manchester and people came from all over Lancashire (and Cheshire) to attend them.

The Manchester Grammar School examination was a frightening experience. There were approximately 1,000 entrants (for 150 places) and I remember sitting in this huge hall surrounded by about 300 other boys. Some boys had done French or Latin at primary (or preparatory) school and they took extra papers in these subjects.

At William Hulme's, by contrast, there were fewer candidates (about 600) for about the same number of places. The examination was over two days and the general knowledge paper took place on the Saturday morning. General knowledge was my forte and I remember writing an authoritative essay on irrigation (my source was the Boys Own Paper!) and trying to draw a wheelbarrow (I have no artistic skills at all!).

My father had taken the preparations for these examinations very seriously indeed, to the extent that he had sent me to a private cramming academy for a period of three months. Hofmann's academy was geared to getting boys (and girls) through the Scholarship as the Eleven Plus was known locally. Mr Hofmann was a Viennese Jew who, having escaped from the Nazis, had set up his school on the Valley, a road that ran up by the side of Boggart Hole Clough from the Tram Office to Moston Lane. There, in a large Victorian bow-windowed house, he drummed the 3Rs into recalcitrant Mancunians. I was afraid of him! A tall commanding presence with a shock of white hair and piercing blue eyes, he hectored us in heavily accented English. I was glad to escape, though no doubt spending this money made my father feel better but I doubt whether it made a scrap of difference to the eventual outcome!

Then came a period of waiting from mid February to late May (and early June). It must have been a difficult time for my parents but with my usual insouciance, I forgot about the whole business. Then the results came in thick and fast; North Manchester High School for Boys (Passed); Manchester Grammar School (Passed; no Scholarship); William Hulme's Grammar School (offered Scholarship; fees plus £100 a year until Higher School Certificate).

At the Avenue Primary School there was a celebration. Mr Dunne summoned everybody to the Hall and we came up to the platform in rank order. I was second after a very bright girl who was to go to Manchester

High school for Girls, the sister school to the Manchester Grammar school. Each one of us was clapped onto the stage as we came up; approximately 25% of the candidates who had sat the examination. The sheep had been separated from the goats! In later years, I thought how humiliating for the goats who were consigned to Domett Street Secondary Modern (and a similar girls' school).

It also sounded the death knell for Our Gang, as we were split up into: me (who went on to a fee-paying school), others who went to North Manchester High School for Boys, and the residue who went to Domett Street. One or two managed to escape from this last institution later, at the age of thirteen years, when they transferred to the Technical College and took up subjects such as metalwork, woodwork, basic draughtsmanship and rubber technology.

When all my results came in, my father, who was pleased with my performance overall, was presented with a dilemma. Should I accept the Scholarship at William Hulme's Grammar School or the place at MGS? After several days of agitation my father decided that we would have to consult Uncle Willie, a momentous step indeed!

Willie was my father's eldest brother, an icon in the family. After service in the Flying Corps, he had joined the Customs Service and became eventually the Senior Customs Officer in the Bonded Warehouse at Salford Docks. He had also progressed to his own semi-detached villa in Urmston which he was buying on a mortgage, a venture previously unknown to the Lee family! Willie was one of that vanished breed, an autodidact. His brothers James, Jack, Harry and Eric, deferred to him; his sisters Bertha and Amy respected him deeply. He was a senior steward of the local Methodist Church and a lifelong teetotaller. An amateur philosopher, his aphorisms have come down through the family: 'People not things'; 'Worse things have happened at sea!'

Having made our appointment with Willie we made as a family our long journey to Urmston in South Manchester – two slow bus journeys in those days. The oracle was in a very good humour! His next-door neighbour, a Christian Scientist, had fallen in his garden, two weeks earlier, had refused treatment and been in agony with a broken fibula. Eventually he had abandoned the power of prayer and had to have Plaster of Paris instead! This appealed to Willie's mischievous sense of humour (a Lee characteristic).

Willie, father and I sat in the front parlour while the situation was outlined to him. After some deliberation he advised my father that I should go to the Grammar School rather than William Hulme's. This decision may have been helped by the fact that Willie already had one son at the Grammar School and another was to follow later. There is nothing like believing in your own decisions!

However the die was cast; Alea jacta est! My father went straight home and wrote the appropriate letters. I was enrolled at the Manchester Grammar School to start in the first week of September 1946. It was to prove a major turning point and there I was to meet my first giant.

CHAPTER 7

Manchester Grammar School and Sir Eric James (1946-1953)

The difference between good teachers and great teachers: good teachers make the best of a pupil's means; great teachers foresee a pupil's ends.

Maria Callas 1923-1977
to Kenneth Harris

INITIALLY THERE WAS to be a disappointment. A letter arrived at Tweedale in early August, to say that I should start at Sale High School for Boys in September. This did not make sense to me but father explained that this school was a preparatory school for the 'Big School' in Rusholme Manchester and I would be there for only two years. The preparatory school uniform was subtly different from that of Big School in that although we still wore the owl (Minerva's fowl for wisdom) – the quarter colours on the cap were yellow (and not blue).

The other problem was to find the school! It involved another family trip: first the 60 bus to Corporation Street then a walk to London Road Station; then onto the electric train and down past Warwick Road (and the cricket ground again) and across the Mersey into Cheshire. Getting off at Brooklands Road we walked half a mile up to the preparatory school which stood desolate and unoccupied on this Sunday in August. I thought what a long way to go to school but later on I would come to enjoy it.

My parents bought me an annual railway contract and so, suitably attired in blazer, cap and tie, loaded down with a heavy satchel, I set off one bright shining morning in September. Soon the litany of the timetable was burnt into my brain: English; French; Arithmetic; Algebra; Geometry; Music (Singing); Physical Education; Handicraft; Geography; and History. The School was divided into four Houses: New (to which I was allocated); Sandbach; Easson; and Atkinson. Our colour was yellow.

In some ways this was inspired, as it replaced old gang loyalties with new ones and to a degree stopped bullying of the younger boys by older ones.

However there was the initiation 'ceremony'. On the first day of term all new boys were to be bumped at the first break (or at lunchtime). This involved four older boys picking up the new boy by the arms and legs and bumping him heavily on the ground three times and shouting 'Bumped'. This was fairly painful but I endured my ordeal as stoically as was possible. You must not, at all costs, break down into tears. It was possible to be attacked twice by mistake and you had to shout, 'Bumped' to try and avoid this.

So the term started and I was introduced to the competitive element of the school. There were tests all the time, terminal examinations and written reports. From the age of eleven, to the age of twenty-six years, when I took the London Membership Examination (for the Royal College of Physicians), I was to become like an examination machine, finely tuned to soak up information like a sponge, and then to regurgitate it in suitable boluses. Fortunately one of my greatest attributes is an excellent memory verging at times on the photographic and this was to prove crucial in the upcoming academic steeplechase.

I can still remember the content of some of those first year lessons, in particular those in History and Geography. In History we studied the Wars of the Roses with the Red versus the White, battles, knights, castles and sieges. In Geography for some reason we started off with the Agricultural Revolution and the great pioneers including Jethro Tull, 'Turnip' Townshend and Coke of Holkham. I became somewhat knowledgeable about the rotation of crops, the fallow period and the fertilizing effect of growing alfalfa and the Leguminosae (peas and beans).

There were two main non-academic activities in these first two years: football and trainspotting. Football was important and I used to emulate Charlie Mitten on the left wing for New House. We managed to win the House Championship twice and on one occasion I scored four goals but three were ruled offside, much to my annoyance as there was no linesman! Later I played for the school team in Under 14 matches against local schools like Altrincham Grammar, Cheadle Hulme, Withington and so on. We were usually soundly beaten but on one occasion we beat a St Bede's team, which included Matt Busby's son, 1-0, which gave us a great fillip!

Most of our surplus energy was concentrated on trainspotting. This was 1946 and the steam trains were still operating in the old liveries of the London Midland and Scottish (LMS) and the London North Eastern (LNER); red and green respectively. The LMS we called the Hell of a Mess and the LNER the Decrepit and Disabled. There were supporters of both who travelled to see the great expresses.

Our first excursion was from Manchester Central to Hartford in Cheshire which lay on the West Coast Main Line, the pride of the LMS. Here, between Warrington and Crewe we would wait on Hartford station, or a mile on the north side, and record trains of the Patriot Class or the Coronation Scot Class going through at almost 100 miles per hour. Regular excursions were made to Hartford as our first haul had been so satisfactory. Sometimes we would put a penny on the line to recover it later in a highly battered state – a most dangerous practice. On another occasion we arrived to find the whole area shrouded in fog and watched with rapt attention as the linesman put detonators on the track and the expresses crept through at 15 mph to the accompaniment of a volley of bangs. To see an express emerge from the fog, get a brief glimpse of the nameplate and find that it was a new 'spot' and could be underlined in the book was an unforgettable experience!

Eventually we were banned from the embankment at Hartford so we decided to go further afield. An LNER enthusiast suggested we go to Doncaster and after much searching through timetables (which we loved) we went from Manchester London Road to Sheffield, and then changed for Doncaster. Donc (or D'Caster), as it was known, was to the LNER aficionados what Crewe was to the LMS. There we waited on the platform, as the 'Streaks' came through, some on a non-stop run from London (Kings Cross) to Edinburgh (Waverley) pulling the Pullman trains. Many of the locomotives were the famous streamlined Gresley Pacifics and when they came through Doncaster at top speed the whole station seemed to shake. On one occasion we saw Mallard the holder of the speed record come through pulling the 10 a.m. from Kings Cross and the three of us jumped round the station platform like dancing dervishes much to the puzzlement of bored travellers.

In 1948 came the nationalization of the railways. The LMS and LNER disappeared, together with their respective liveries, to be replaced by the boring British Railways (BR). We were disgusted! By coincidence we

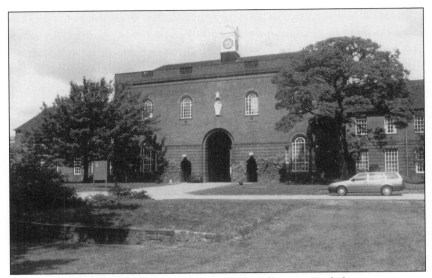

Manchester Grammar School; Old Hall Lane, Rusholme.

moved that year to the main School in Rusholme and stopped travelling on the train anyway. Even to this day however, if I see a steam locomotive, I am transported back to Hartford and Doncaster over fifty years ago!

Our class was divided when we were transferred to Rusholme. The top four went into Upper 3 Modern (U3M) and as I had usually finished second or third this was to be my form (note form not class!). The first impression of the main school was overwhelming because of its sheer size: 1,200 boys, with 400 in the Sixth Form. When the whole number gathered together for Assembly in the morning it had to be seen to be believed. The accompaniment to hymn singing was provided by an organ which could have done good service at one of the great cathedrals.

The High Master, Sir Eric James, would enter for Assembly in his gown followed by fifteen to twenty other masters similarly attired. They climbed onto the platform and he would address us like a large public meeting. Behind him, and the other masters, sat the serried ranks of the choir (about 100 boys). Sir Eric addressed us through a microphone and I can hear his voice in my ear now, 'This is *yer* school and *yer* must look after it' – the '*yer*' was affectation for you but produced an inimitable effect. 'We must seek *culture* with all our efforts. You have been cast into a great heritage; *yer* must be worthy of this heritage. This school has an enviable record of Oxbridge success; I hope the Senior Sixth is aware of this record and will seek to emulate or surpass it'. The sentences come ringing down the years. As will emerge, I saw much more of him later when I reached the Sixth Form and attempted to gain a University place.

Eventually, I was able, with my three colleagues from Sale, to find the form room for U3M (Upper Three Modern). I grabbed a desk at the back and the other form members gathered. They viewed the gang of four from Sale High with suspicion tinged with disdain! However there was no time for discussion as Billy Hulme swept into the room and we rose, as one boy, to greet him. He flung his academic gown onto a chair and glowering at us said, 'Sit!'

Billy Hulme was to be our form master for the next two years and it is necessary to give some account of him. He was somewhat stout, about 5 ft 6 ins in height with a shaven bullet head and glasses. Slightly stooped he ruled by fear and regimentation. The first thing he did was to go round each individual who had to stand up and tell Billy his name, who then either grunted or passed some remark. I said, 'Lee from Sale'.

There was a pause. Billy said, 'Ah, we will have to see how you four get on, as you are something of an unknown quantity'. After this implied threat he then said, 'Have you a relative in the School?' 'Yes,' I replied, 'James Lee in 4C'. James was Uncle Willie's son. Billy replied, 'Well I hope you will do better than him!' and passed on to the next victim.

Billy was to continue our French teaching and to start German from scratch. I had not been particularly keen on French at Sale but German gripped me from the start, particularly if Billy launched into one of his Adolf Hitler speeches, or reminisced about his experiences in the Great War. I struggled with masculine, feminine and neuter; the dative and the accusative but eventually it all began to fall into place. It would pay off many years later in the London MRCP examination!

Billy had peculiar ideas about corporal punishment. He had a collection of large wooden spoons but he did not use these any more. He either used the widely sanctioned gym shoe on the backside or asked the potential victim if he would prefer the punishment to be administered in the school swimming pool.

Once a week he supervised swimming which took place completely in the nude. Billy would administer his punishment with the bare hand applied to the bare buttock. I once received five smacks and with the last stroke there was a slight squeeze of the buttock. Looking back on it, it is probable that as a lifelong bachelor, he favoured male company but as all the Masters had unusual foibles it did not strike us as that peculiar at the time.

It was a very distinguished form: Michael Barber, sadly now dead, a friend of mine at school, became Professor of Chemistry at Manchester and FRS; Walter Bodmer was knighted for his service to genetics and medicine; and there were many others who excelled in later life.

Time moved on. The question arose next, to which section of the Sixth Form should I move after School Certificate? The position was made difficult by the fact that I had overtures from several different directions. First the Maths master wanted me to join their section. This offer was quickly rejected, as though I was competent in the subject, I had no abiding interest. The second offer was much more tempting. I had won the Form History Prize for finishing first in this subject and the History master, Chalmers, pleaded with me to continue into the Sixth Form. I thought long and hard about it but eventually I said to him outright that my first love Medicine (and hence the Biology Sixth) must take precedence. He replied very generously that 'we need good people in Medicine' and I felt extremely flattered.

I therefore entered the Biology Department never having done biology at School Certificate Level. I was to be entered at Higher School Certificate level in Zoology, Botany and Chemistry. The Biology Department was separated physically from the rest of the school and comprised two classrooms, two large laboratories and a greenhouse (of which more later). My form was now 61BZ literally the first year of the Botanical/Zoological Sixth. The three masters were Minns (Zoology), Speight (Botany) and Davies (General Biology). We went to the Chemistry Department to Mr Hicks for tuition in this subject.

If Billy Hulme had been somewhat unusual then Mr Minns and Mr Speight were distinctly eccentric! Mr Minns wore usually a dishevelled brown suit, with his tie all awry, and carried a broken old briefcase. He dragged one leg (probably old polio) and talked in a very 'cut glass' accent. Our hypothesis was that he was the illegitimate son of a baronet but we had no definite evidence for this hypothesis! He drove a battered old Alvis and those who had visited his home said he had a six-foot Buddha in his front room.

Mr Speight by contrast was 6 ft tall and immaculately dressed. His knowledge of botany and plant identification was encyclopaedic. He really should have been a University Lecturer as he hated boys and tried to avoid them as far as possible. He was the constant butt of practical jokes which included variously; blocking his car in with a mammoth snowball; binding and gagging one of the boys (a future Professor of Bacteriology) and rolling him into a classroom in front of the astonished master; and burning the cacti in the departmental greenhouse with cigarettes!

The greenhouse was nominally under Mr Speight's direction and he waged a constant battle to preserve the plants. When he was away at lunch we used to turn the sprinklers on or close all the windows on sunny days. We were very unkind to him at the time but enjoyed every minute of it. It leavened the hard grind of academic work as the form settled down.

Sir Eric James now came into the day to day scene. A chemist by trade, he had obtained a postgraduate degree in the subject. He now intimated to Mr Hicks that he would give us a few lessons in Organic Chemistry. These were a tour de force! He swept into the classroom like a God descending from Mount Olympus and began to despatch the thunder-bolts of Jove. In one particular lesson, he covered the whole blackboard with symbols, end groups and arrows and announced, at the end of 45 minutes, that he had done the whole of the syllabus and we simply had to be able to reproduce this map. He then swept out as though with 'a puff of blue smoke'.

He also gave us a short course of Philosophy lectures which included Plato, Aristotle, Locke, Rousseau, Bentham and Mill and introduced concepts such as the Noble Savage and Utilitarianism. We listened slack jawed to these performances. In his last address he concluded 'You must not be narrow technocrats but familiar with philosophy, music and literature. Only then will you be able to serve *yer* country as men of the New Enlightenment'. It was no surprise to any of us when later on he was chosen to initiate, as Vice-Chancellor, the new University at York.

Eventually the examinations came and the results followed. I had obtained Distinctions in all three subjects. Mr Minns wrote to say that these should guarantee me a State Scholarship and they did. Thereby there would be a place in a suitable University to read Medicine. Mr

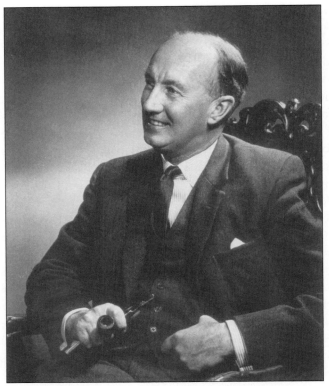

Eric James, High Master of Manchester Grammar School.
Later Lord James of Rusholme.

Minns strongly advised me not to take the place I had been offered at Manchester University but to return for a third year in the Sixth Form and try for Oxford or Cambridge. This, after some discussion with my parents, I decided to do; my father somewhat reluctantly surrendering long held visions of my entering Owens College.

Matters were now complicated by my falling in love. I had had several girlfriends since the age of sixteen but no relationship had lasted more than two or three months. This was to be very different. I met Kathleen!

I had been vaguely conscious of girls in green uniforms travelling with us towards Rusholme and Whalley Range on the 53 bus. One day I spotted Kathleen and Cupid's arrow struck! She was sixteen at the time with a mass of black hair; blue eyes and nicely turned ankles. By judicious enquiries I found that, to my delight, she lived in Blackley. Very shortly afterwards I introduced myself and a relationship started that was to last for six years. She was a Roman Catholic and was attending St Joseph's College in Whalley Range where she was studying shorthand, typing, English and so on.

Initially the relationship was Platonic but eventually it became emotional and passionate. I had to fall back on my knowledge of the 'safe period'. There were some benefits in learning about the details of the menstrual cycle for Higher Zoology after all! At this time there was no such thing as the oral contraceptive or the 'morning after' pill! Eventually in the late summer of 1952 my parents became aware that something was going on. When challenged I had to admit that I was going out with a Roman Catholic. My father was mortified and a series of blinding rows ensued. I flatly refused to give up Kathleen and as I was eighteen my father could hardly make me do so. Her parents were aware of the hostility and this made the situation doubly difficult as she was exhorted to find 'a good Catholic boy'. I was genuinely in love with Kathleen but part of the trouble also, I am sure, was my anti-authoritarian stance and the syndrome of the old stag (father) versus the young stag (me). At all events, I lived in a state of sullen hostility with regard to my father for a number of years. I decided to find out about Roman Catholicism and used to attend Mass whilst on holiday with Kathleen in Ireland and also to study the Missal regularly.

I returned to school in September 1952 to be appointed a prefect and to be summoned to a council of war by the Senior Chemistry Master Mr Plackett who supervised the assault on Oxford and Cambridge. Every year each sixth former who had stayed on at school was given a plan of action. Mine went as follows: 'You will enter the Closed Scholarships for Brasenose Oxford in October; failing that you will go for Magdalen Oxford in the Open Scholarships in December; failing that Christ's Cambridge in January; and the last chance is at St Catherine's or Selwyn at Cambridge in April'. I had no idea where any of these colleges were but to quote Tennyson 'their's not to reason why, their's but to do and die'.

The first hurdle was the Brasenose closed examination, which about eight of us attempted, sat in a small room at school. I remember discussing the oxides of iron and commenting on the question 'Are parasites degenerate?' There was also a general paper which included such questions as 'What is the value of Tradition?' and we were asked to write an essay on Revenge, Retribution and Forgiveness.

A few weeks passed and then I was summoned to Brasenose for interview. Here Sir Eric James played an important part, telling me to feature as my interests football (for a local church); Mozart (Einer Kleiner Nacht-Musik and Die Zauberflöte) and collecting insects (I had just found a devil's coach horse beetle). 'Tod' Sweet and I travelled up to a foggy Oxford on a dismal November day. Sir Eric knew his dons very well and one of them became animated when I told him about my interest in Mozart, using the German pronunciation. Finally one of the Fellows turned to me and said 'Is it really true that Dr James teaches you Plato in the Sixth Form?' This was like a leg stump full toss and I dispatched it over the boundary rope for six, as I had been reading my philosophy notes on the train!

Tod and I returned to Manchester and within 48 hours, I received a call to go to the High Master's Office where he greeted me with an outstretched hand and said 'Lee. Congratulations! You have been awarded the Somerset Thornhill Scholarship at Brasenose'. He sat me down and went over the details of the interview questions as he liked to know what the dons were thinking. He was particularly interested in the question about Plato and philosophy. 'They think it's all a stunt,' he said, 'but it isn't'. He also told me that my General paper had been poor and gave me a reading list for the next few months. I walked out of the office on a cloud. I could hardly believe it – from the back streets of Manchester to Brasenose College Oxford. It seemed incredible! I showed the contents of the award envelope to Kathleen on the bus home. She was very pleased for me but I think we both recognized that the enforced separation might lead to a break-up. For the moment we had all of nine months to enjoy.

I also recognized that, in Eric James, I had met an intellectual giant. He was the first in my odyssey and I shall never forget him. He advised me, at our final interview, that I should go to St Mary's Hospital, Paddington for my clinical training. I did not realize then that Pickering was at St Mary's at that time (1953) and it was his unit that James was recommending. I was indeed to meet (and work for) Pickering, but not at St Mary's London but at the Radcliffe Infirmary in Oxford some ten years later.

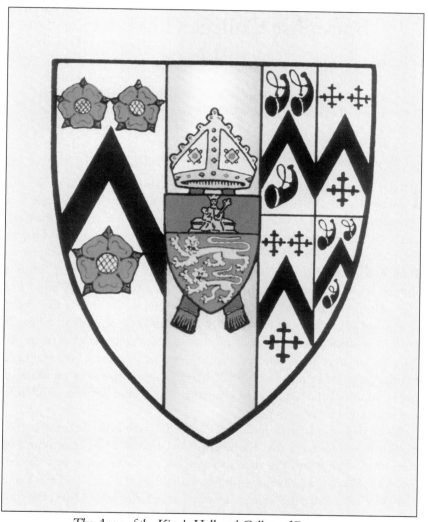

The Arms of the King's Hall and College of Brasenose.

CHAPTER 8

Brasenose College (1953-1956)

When you go to the University let it be Oxford rather than
Cambridge for two reasons: because Oxford has far the better air
and in Brazennose College there are many peculiar privileges in
favour of Lancashire men.

Edward Moore
1667.

I HAD NEVER HEARD of Brasenose College until I went there for the
interview in 1952. Founded in 1508 the name of the College is a
corruption of Brass Nose. A great brass nose in the form of a knocker
hangs on the front door to this day. On one occasion the monks who ran
the College fell out with the University authorities and decamped to
Stamford in Lincolnshire. They were persuaded to return later! Famous
alumni include the distinguished author John Buchan (of *Thirty Nine
Steps* fame) and Bishop Heber of Calcutta who wrote the hymn 'From
Greenland's icy mountains to India's coral strand'. Generally the college is
more cosmopolitan than some and, in my day, drew students from the
North Country, Scotland, and the Old Commonwealth, for example
South Africa, Australia, and New Zealand. There was also a tradition of
rugby and cricket players, thus ensuring a good mix between academic
and sporting activities.

When I arrived there in October 1953 I was both homesick (for
Blackley) and lovesick (for Kathleen). I have never been enamoured of
communal living and the first two years were to be spent in College.
'Staircase Seven top; sharing with Stockdale' said the porter in the lodge
that faces onto Radcliffe Square. I went through the main Quad, past the
famous sundial and into the back Quad. There was staircase VII with its
Roman numeral. I trudged up the stair with my heavy suitcase and
knocked on the door. In I went and there was Neville Stockdale with
whom I was to share this set of rooms for the next year. Neville was to
prove a delightful companion for the next period of time. A tall well-built

son of Keighley in West Yorkshire, he came to be known to us as the 'Big Yorkshireman'. He was to study chemistry. We shared a common sitting room and off this there were two separate bedrooms. We soon got a kettle and tea-making apparatus and settled down to domestic bliss.

All meals were taken in the Hall. In the evening we had to don our gowns: long for me (scholar) and short for Neville (commoner), and go down at seven o'clock to the dimly lit room. We sat for a moment (or two) and then in came the Principal and Fellows. We rose and then sat down again. The Organ Scholar said the shortest grace he could find which was usually, 'Benedictus benedicat' and the meal commenced!

The next thing was to arrange to see the Fellow and Tutor in Physiology, Dr George Gordon. After one evening meal, I waited on a gloomy cold staircase for the man to arrive. Eventually this tall, angular, bespectacled figure came up at a fast pace. He turned out to be a shy individual and initially the tutorials proved to be painful as I also was inhibited had not yet learned to think and knew no physiology! I was supposed to read about the structure of the veins and the nature of the venous pulse. This was impenetrable initially but, by happy chance, rooting round in the BNC library, I found an American textbook by Wiggers called *The Cardiovascular System*. The situation was transformed! My relationship with Dr Gordon began to prosper.

Another stroke of good fortune was that my colleague from the Sixth Form, at MGS, Nigel Keddie, had won a Scholarship to Oriel College to read medicine. He was accommodated in a room in Oriel Street just across the High from BNC. He became my partner in anatomy and thus started a relationship which would last for eight years and take us through to qualification in medicine and beyond. Nigel and I presented a common front to the outside world but between the two of us was a long lasting intense competition which acted to our mutual benefit.

The first serious hurdle in our course was anatomy. Anatomy: the very word rings like a tocsin in the memories of medical students of our era. We had, in a short two years, to dissect the whole of the human body; to study the nerves, blood vessels and lymphatics and the detailed structure of the tissues (histology). It was, in retrospect, a fearsome task. Every fortnight we had a viva voce examination and could not proceed to the next part until this test had been negotiated satisfactorily. Dealing with corpses, whole and dismembered, did not bother us one jot, as one session followed another. We cheerfully sluiced the human fat off our hands at lunchtime and dashed back to College, ate a hearty meal and started off again in the afternoon. The leg was followed by the arm; the head and neck; the abdomen and the thorax; five terms of intense effort followed by a term for revision.

On one occasion we smuggled Neville Stockdale into the dissection room early in the morning. He had never seen a dead body so we showed him a few. Fortunately he did not pass out (and was not challenged) or we would have found ourselves in trouble under the provisions of the Anatomy Act 1832!

Nigel wanted to be a surgeon and was a fine anatomist. He subsequently carried off the Theodore Williams Scholarship in this subject. I regarded it simply as a means to an end as I wanted to find out about rheumatic fever, pernicious anaemia and Vitamin B12! I was therefore very pleased when the lectures on the Vitamins appeared at the end of the first year.

As far as College life was concerned this involved two main activities, playing cards, usually cribbage, in our rooms and heavy drinking in the town. When you release a group of eighteen year olds into the streets of Oxford, away from parental control, there is bound to be experimentation with drink and a temptation to excessive consumption. The first discovery was the Junior Common Room at the College and its buttery. This was basically a pub with its own lounge bar and vault. Before, or after, the evening meal we would gather in there to sup the College ale. One of the men could play Jelly Roll Morton piano rags on the Joanna and here was started my lifetime interest in traditional jazz. The College servants (or scouts) would also gather after their day's duties were over, and we were expected to buy them a pint (or two) which we duly did.

We also explored other hostelries in the neighbourhood including the Chequers, the Eagle and Child (Bird and Baby), The Trout at Godstow and so on. We used to stagger back to College where we had to be in by midnight or the great doors would be closed.

On several occasions in those first two years we missed the witching hour and had to 'climb in'. This involved a well-known and tested route. Down into the Turl, a street off the High, and then over the wall into the garden belonging to the Rector of Lincoln College was the first stage. Then you had to crawl across the garden on all fours, under his drawing

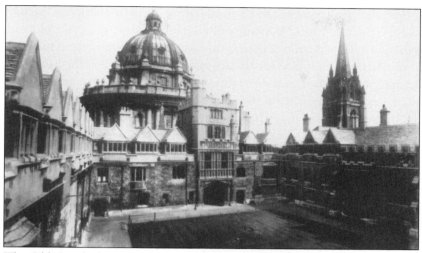

The Old Quad of Brasenose. Beyond the gatehouse, on the left, is the Radcliffe Camera and, on the right, St Mary's University Church. A suitable refuge for Lancashire men!

room window, to the wall which was the boundary between Lincoln and BNC. Then the difficult part came, which was to get over this wall and onto the roof of the bicycle sheds. This roof was made of corrugated iron sections and if you came down on it with too much force there was a tremendous racket! A Senior Fellow of BNC, Robert Shackleton, had his rooms immediately above this area so it was important to make sure that his curtains were drawn. Then the last stage was to climb carefully down one of the stanchions of the bicycle shed and move quickly into one of the outside toilets where you would wait to make sure that you had not been seen (or heard) and the coast was clear. The safe haven of Staircase VII was then very close. Occasionally someone fell on (or off) the bicycle sheds and Dr Shackleton (and the porters) would apprehend them and they would be fined and gated for a period!

Apart from these amateur efforts the College had a serious climbing club which assailed the Radcliffe Camera and the Codrington Library of All Souls College, where chamber pots were hung on the pinnacles! However a member of this unofficial group was killed climbing in Snowdonia in our first year, and this cast a definite gloom over the College for a number of weeks.

The first two years of the medical course passed remarkably quickly
and the Anatomy and Physiology examinations were upon us. All I can
remember about them is writing a thirty-minute essay on the rectum and
in the Anatomy viva being handed a patella (knee cap) and the hoary old
question being asked, is it the right or left? You put it down on the table
and the way it tilts gives you the right answer!

Nigel and I passed the examination with flying colours and now had to
find 'digs' or lodgings for the 3rd or Honours Year in Physiology. Neville
Stockdale would join his friend Chris Lupton in lodgings off the Cowley
Road but we ended up at 69 Morrell Avenue, on a road leading up to
Headington Hill. This was to prove to be an inspired choice as Mrs Bate
our landlady was a treasure. She had been widowed at an early age when
her husband died from pulmonary tuberculosis (TB) and she had been
left to bring up two small children which she had done very successfully.
Now she had become the epitome of the Oxford landlady with her cheery
burr and the massive traditional English breakfasts that she cooked for us.
We had to pay extra for baths; the hot water being provided by an Ascot
heater. The house was very cold in the severe Oxford winter that
followed and for a couple of weeks I slept in my dressing gown. Nevertheless it was most welcome to move away from the collegiate communal
living.

The third year was made up of sections of General, Neuro and
Respiratory Physiology together with oceans of Biochemistry. George
Gordon summoned me and said that I was to be 'farmed out' to J.R.P.
O'Brien (Percy), at Pembroke College, for tutorials in Biochemistry. This
was to be an experience in itself! He conducted his tutorials at his large
house in North Oxford, usually at 8 p.m. in the evening, after dinner.
When my first essay had been submitted, to my surprise he politely
offered me a glass of sherry and then set about my essay (and me) with
the proverbial flame-thrower. He said, 'the facts are here but it is as dull
as ditchwater. You are capable of getting first class honours but you will
have to pull your socks up!' I staggered out of his house an hour and a
half later and realized that this was very different from my gentlemanly
exchanges with George Gordon and would require my full attention!
Percy and I battled with each other for the full eight weeks and I would
have called it an honourable draw. I was summoned to Responsions
(assessments) in the College Hall at the end of term in front of the

Principal, Senior Tutor and the Fellows, to review my progress. A letter from Percy was read out which, summarized, said, 'Lee has every prospect of gaining first class honours and I am sure he will do so if he continues to work at the present rate for the next six months'. I was staggered! The Principal, Platnauer, looked at me rather quizzically and said, 'We have come to rely on Dr O'Brien's opinion. Keep up the good work'. As I left the Hall, I began to realize that Percy's brusque combative approach had helped me to think and marshall an argument. How helpful this would prove to be when I tried desperately in later years to become a clinical scientist.

The months moved on inexorably and piles of papers accumulated at 69 Morrell Avenue. We worked a 9 a.m. to 9 p.m. day with approximately five hours in the Radcliffe Science Library. Meals were snatched hastily: lunch often in the College, supper in the Municipal Restaurant just over Magdalen Bridge, an occasional game of snooker and then straight back to the Library. I occasionally used to hide volumes in the stacks, to thwart competitors and in order to retrieve them after supper! At long last the Physiology Finals came after a frenzied period of revision. We donned our academic subfusc: dark suit, winged collar, white bow tie and mortar-board. Mrs Bate in a kindly gesture gave Nigel and me a rose from the garden for our buttonholes and off we went to the Examination Schools on our bicycles. It was the end of the beginning!

The written papers went very well but the practical examinations were a nightmare. I have never been very good with my hands and this, allied with a lack of depth perception resulting from my eye injury, gave me severe problems. I struggled through the six hour Biochemistry Practical and the final morning was confronted with George Gordon (the BNC tutor) over a preparation in the frog of the sciatic nerve/gastrocnemius muscle. He asked me a series of unanswerable questions. I was glad to flee the room, join Nigel and make the railway journey back to Manchester.

That evening I phoned Nigel from a local call box, who said that we had both obtained 1st Class Honours. Evidently Mrs Bate had gone down to the Schools, after she had finished work, looked at the list, which had gone up at 5 p.m. She had found our names in the First Division, to her delight and surprise, and somehow let Nigel know, as he was on the telephone and 24 Tweedale was not. It turned out that 69 Morrell Avenue had half of the 1st Class Honours Degrees awarded that year in Physiology!

I slept continuously for about a fortnight as I was absolutely exhausted. I was then able to re-establish my relationship with Kathleen, much to my father's annoyance, and to consider the future. Nigel and I had been given a provisional place at the Manchester University clinical school provided we had 'satisfied' the examiners at Oxford. I was in bed one morning at Tweedale at 10 a.m. when Nigel turned up in his Ford Anglia (he was now driving). 'Get dressed; we have to go and see the Dean, Dr Brockbank, at Manchester.' It turned out that we both had been awarded Entrance Clinical Scholarships and were to start clinical medicine the following day! This after only a fortnight's holiday.

The rest of that week was a blur as we registered and found that we were to be attached to M3 ward at the Manchester Royal Infirmary under the aegis of Dr William Brockbank, Dean of the Medical School and Consultant Physician. I rushed round and bought a stethoscope, a Queen's Square reflex hammer and a Keeler ophthalmoscope as badges of my new office. I was to be a doctor!

CHAPTER 9

Manchester University and Douglas Black (1956-1959)

Mark what ills the scholar's life assail,
Toil, envy, want the patron and the jail.
Dr Samuel Johnson
1709-1784
The Vanity of Human Wishes

A GROUP OF EIGHT of us arrived on M3 ward that mid-July morning. This was to be 'walking the wards', as the old descriptions had it. I had never felt so gauche and embarrassed in my life. Fortunately, in the first stages, we practised history taking and physical examination on each other and not on the patients. We gradually learned the rote of 'Inspection; palpation; percussion; and auscultation'. Having, as I described, acquired a stethoscope, a Queen's Square reflex hammer and a Keeler wide-angle ophthalmoscope, I practised assiduously. This last instrument, even though I could only use it with my left eye, was to prove an ever present help in trouble and, as we shall see, took me right through to the Membership Examination of the College of Physicians.

Clinical medicine was so vast and we were so small, figuratively speaking, that it was overwhelming. The big textbooks of medicine like Price and Cecil were 2,000 pages long. Our mentors encouraged us; it would all fall into place eventually. I can still remember several of the patients: a lady with ulcerative colitis who was very kind to me in my amateurish fumblings; an old man with coal gas poisoning who was cherry red; another old man who suffering from acute pyelonephritis developed febrile rigors which shook his cot-sided bed across the floor and were accompanied by body temperatures of 104°F (in old money!).

The mornings were spent on M3M and M3F, the male and female wards (shepherded by the kind Dr Brockbank). The afternoons were devoted to 'Bugs and Drugs', as it was known affectionately. This

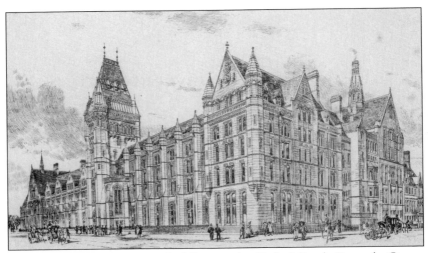

Manchester University main building on the Oxford Road. Formerly Owens College; this is a late nineteenth century engraving.

comprised Pathology; Bacteriology; Virology; and Pharmacology. We had to attend post-mortems at 8 a.m. in the morning. My two abiding memories of these early starts were first one of the pathologists removing the top of the cranium with an electric saw, to expose the brain and cranial cavity; and second entering the post-mortem room one morning to an overwhelming stench of decay and corruption emanating from the abdominal contents of a corpse; the individual had died of septic peritonitis.

We plugged away at all these studies gradually eroding our mountains of ignorance and learning to stitch, set up an intravenous drip and do lumbar punctures. Occasionally we were allowed to assist in theatre and I was hopeless in this regard largely because I was effectively one-eyed. Cutting sutures was a nightmare as I could not see what I was doing!

The most dramatic part of the Clinical course was Practical Midwifery. There were two four-week sessions in this; at St Mary's Hospital in Central Manchester and at Withington Hospital on the south side of the city. Obstetrics involved hours (or days) of hanging about followed by bursts of frenzied activity. We were supposed to do twenty normal deliveries and had to compete with the trainee midwives to obtain our quota. This led to tensions both within and outside our camp. We had to learn how to deliver the head; then the rest of the body, clamp and cut the cord; and then finally deal with the placenta. We whiled away the time by playing snooker waiting for these normal deliveries.

On one occasion I nearly 'passed out'. We were summoned at 3 a.m. by the Resident Surgical Officer. It was an awful case: a woman had suffered a respiratory arrest at another hospital and was brought into St Mary's with the baby still in utero. There was no foetal monitoring in those days but the baby's heart could not be heard. The Resident Surgical Officer applied the forceps to the baby's head and by brute force pulled the infant out. Of course it was dead. We, as a group, had been stood on a dais at the back of the theatre watching events. I began feeling a little sick and a little dizzy. Fortunately, I realized I was going to faint and retreated from the operating theatre and collapsed onto my bed where I slept until morning. I was to see many other gruesome sights in the course of the next three years but this was the only one that lowered my blood pressure!

The next stage of Obstetrics was to go on the district with the local (or travelling) midwife. This involved visiting for home deliveries some of the dilapidated properties of Inner Manchester at Longsight, Moss Side and Whalley Range. The memories here are kaleidoscopic but it was an eventful period. One mother went mad (puerperal psychosis); another had a post partum haemorrhage and went with the Flying Squad to St Mary's; another caused me my most embarrassing clinical experience.

I arrived, shortly after the District Midwife, to find a woman having a precipitate delivery. I hung onto the head but the desire to push was so great that baby came out at express speed together with a vast volume of liquor fluid heavily stained with meconium (intestinal contents). Most of this foul smelling meconium went onto my trousers which were saturated and stinking! I got back to the residence as soon as I could and disposed of the trousers via the hospital incineration system. I then had a bath from head to toe and sent the rest of my clothes to be laundered. My fellow students laughed their heads off in the grim, sardonic way that bespeaks the carapace that we were developing to cope with the slings and arrows of outrageous fortune.

Our final midwifery attachment was at Withington Hospital where, being bored out of our minds one night, some of us went down to the Red Lion pub in the village. Having consumed several pints of bitter we got into the Nurses' Home and persuaded several of them to join us, in our residence. We then held an impromptu party which was absolutely against the rules! The next day those of us who had been involved, realizing that there would be a 'stink', left the course (it was coming to an end anyway) and went on holiday! As a result, my name was to bear a Red Triangle in the records for the rest of the clinical course. I did my best thereafter to avoid trouble!

As we progressed through the years of training I began to consider what I would do on qualifying. Certain subjects were eliminated without a moment's thought: Surgery (couldn't do it); Obstetrics (drama and mess); Pathology (post-mortems). Other parts had more appeal, General Practice (contact with patients); Psychiatry (but frightening); Paediatrics (but nappies and squalling kids) and finally General Medicine.

My mind was finally made up when I was exposed to the work of the University Department of Medicine which comprised amongst others Douglas Black (Professor), Bill Stanbury (Senior Lecturer) and Geoffrey Berlyne (Clinical Tutor). They gave us a course of lectures on the kidney, and I was fascinated. Douglas Black was dry and witty, speaking about sodium and potassium; Bill Stanbury ebullient on calcium and phosphate metabolism; and Geoffrey Berlyne stimulating on acute and chronic renal failure.

When I had been at Oxford, I had read the great American physiologist Homer Smith and his book on the kidney and I realized that the work of the Manchester group was, in many ways, an extension of Smith's physiological principles into medical practice.

I approached Professor Black and told him I intended to imitate him and seek a job in his Department, following qualification, in order that I might do fundamental research on the kidney. He looked mildly surprised but in his customary dry way said that although this was a laudable objective, I should walk before I tried to run. I must qualify first and then go on and obtain the Membership examination of the Royal College of Physicians. This latter qualification was a sine qua non for progression up the medical ladder. Somewhat deflated I returned to catheterizing old men in Senior Surgery and weighing babies in Paediatrics! However, I would meet Douglas Black again when I became his house physician later. In my spare time, I read his book on sodium metabolism and Thompson and King's treatise on Biochemistry in Relation to Medicine. This I regarded as necessary preparation for my distinguished career in renal and

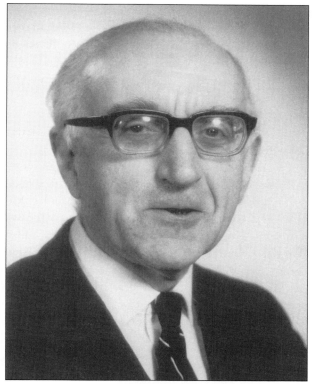

Douglas Andrew Kilgour Black (1913-2002). One-time Professor of Medicine at the University of Manchester; later President of the Royal College of Physicians of London.

metabolic medicine! In the preface to his book Douglas quoted the Red Queen in Alice in Wonderland: 'It takes all one's running to keep in the same place'. I was certainly running very hard at this stage! I fastened on to good bedside teachers of clinical medicine including Stretton and Leonard and they helped me a great deal. Christmas 1958 approached and there were just six months to go to Finals.

My relationship with Kathleen, of six years standing, ended in a blazing row. It had gone on too long without me being able to offer her any prospects of a secure future. Also as tension mounted in the medical course, my behaviour towards her became unreasonable. I always react badly to periods of uncertainty and heavy work. I regretted our split immediately but the breach could not be repaired. I followed this, in early 1959, with a bout of influenza which left me depressed and shortly after that developed bacterial cystitis and had to go and see Dr Jelenowicz, our family doctor, who gave me a course of sulphonamides. He asked after my mother and then said, 'what are you going to do when you qualify?' The burning question of the time.

I remained apathetic as Finals approached. It was what was called a Big Bang Final with Medicine, Surgery, Obstetrics, Gynaecology and Paediatrics all in together.

Nigel and I journeyed to Oxford and stayed with his old Scout in Oriel Street. We prepared for the coming fortnight. Strangely I had no fear of not passing – I felt that the outcome was inevitable! As a result, apart from some rustiness in the opening paper, I sailed through the whole thing diagnosing variously bronchiectasis; aortic incompetence; mitral stenosis; carcinoma of the colon; Devic's disease (neuromyelitis optica); and Rhesus incompatibility. Apart from hurting a patient with the vaginal speculum, with my usual hamfistedness, everything was absolutely straightforward.

I appeared for the first of the final vivas (Medicine) with Leslie Witts (Nuffield Professor of Medicine) and Campbell of Guys, a cardiologist. I braced myself for a nasty leg break. 'Now Lee', said Witts, 'where did you do your clinical training?' Witts knew the answer already – it was Manchester – but I replied without hesitation, 'The Manchester Royal Infirmary'. A slight smile played over his face – he was a famous graduate of that School. He turned to Dr Campbell and said, 'I have no further questions; Dr Campbell over to you'. I waited for the hand grenade to be lobbed over, such as what are the causes of a green tongue, or give me a short classification of the porphyrias! He looked at me in a kindly almost avuncular fashion and said, 'Who taught you to listen for the aortic diastolic murmur down the left sternal edge in the 3rd interspace?' For a moment I was completely flummoxed as they say in Manchester and then said, 'Crichton Bramwell'. 'Oh', he said, 'A fine cardiologist'. He turned to Witts and said, 'I have no more questions'. In this unusual fashion ended my undergraduate training in medicine.

The final ordeal (of all these ordeals) was the Obstetrics and Gynaecology viva. I stumbled through a series of questions on the gynaecological causes of urinary incontinence, my knowledge of which could have been written in a flowing hand on a postage stamp! The bell rang and the Internal Examiner said, 'Alright, Mr Lee. If you ever want a job in Obstetrics in Oxford just get in touch. You may go'. I staggered out of the office after thanking him. Little did he know that I was glad to see the back of Obstetrics and that my academic knowledge of the subject was simply a means to an end. Figuratively, I wiped the dust off my feet both from Obstetrics and from Oxford. Little did I know that I would be returning to the City of Dreaming Spires within two years!

The Final Examination results would be declared at 2.30 p.m. in the Students' Residence at Osler House close to the Radcliffe Infirmary. I was reasonably confident as none of my vivas in Medicine, Surgery or Obstetrics had been overwhelming. Nigel was worried, as his Obstetrics viva had involved him delivering a manikin through a human pelvis in the breech position (a test indeed).

We approached the Board. M.R. Lee and N.C. Keddie had satisfied the examiners. It was a defining moment and I could hardly believe it. I turned to Nigel and shook his hand. 'Congratulations Dr Keddie', I said, and he reciprocated. I felt in what the psychiatrists call a fugue-like state, which I have only experienced on two occasions since: the day I got married to Judith and the day of my inaugural lecture at Edinburgh University.

Time stood still for the whole of what remained of that day. We booked an evening meal by telephone at a hotel in Warwick, calling ourselves Doctors! The staff of the hotel must have wondered who these two fresh-faced youths were. Nigel drove carefully through the English Midlands and we arrived in Manchester very late in the evening. He dropped me off at Victoria Avenue corner in Higher Blackley and he went on to Oldham. I walked home very slowly: past Hill Lane; past the Avenue Primary School where it had all started; past Hopkinson Road Methodist Chapel and turned into Tweedale Avenue. I opened the front door to see my father sitting in his usual armchair. I stood there for a moment and then said, 'That's it. I'm through!' Within minutes I was in bed. I felt empowered: I had at last found out about rheumatic fever and pernicious anaemia. They had become, in fact, like old friends!

CHAPTER 10

Lancaster and Judith (1959-1960)

Flower o' the broom,
Take away love and our earth is a tomb.
Robert Browning
1812-1889
Fra Lippo Lippi 51

FOR TWO WEEKS I was in a state of euphoria. I informed all the neighbours and anyone else, who cared to listen, that I was now a doctor. My old friends from the Tweedale gang regarded me with a mixture of incredulity and suspicion. I changed my cheque book details and had a telephone installed as a matter of urgency, saying that I was 'on call' at home, which was a downright lie! I also rang up a girl called Monica I was interested in and, getting her mother instead, told her that Dr Lee was enquiring after her. This caused some confusion initially as she did not know a Dr Lee! I then took her out to a very posh hotel in Manchester for dinner.

This Walter Mitty phase lasted for about a fortnight. Nigel and I had to take up posts as pre-registration house surgeons (or house physicians). As the date of declaration of the Oxford results was delayed, compared to those at Manchester, we had to be accommodated elsewhere for our first jobs. The Dean, Dr Brockbank, had kindly arranged that we should go to the Royal Lancaster Infirmary, myself as house surgeon and Nigel as house physician. We were told to report there on the first of August 1959 ready for duty.

On the previous evening we took the train up the main line from Manchester Victoria to Lancaster Castle. As we drew into Lancaster, across the canal, there was the Infirmary on the right and a fellow passenger who had obviously read our luggage labels said, 'There it is'. I was very apprehensive and insecure. Six years training: would it get me through? I did not like and did not intend to pursue surgery. This was just

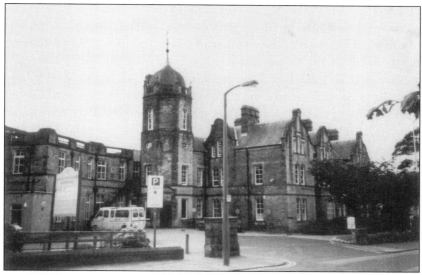

The Royal Lancaster Infirmary.

a means to an end before the 'proper' study of general internal medicine could begin.

I was introduced to the three general surgeons: Mr Hall Drake (an Englishman) and two Scots from the hard-bitten Glasgow School, Magauran and McFadyean. During the day my responsibilities were largely routine: clerking patients, taking blood samples and setting up intravenous and 'cut down' drips. At night it was very different. I was first on call for surgical emergencies which ranged from perforated duodenal ulcer, to acute cholecystitis, to third degree burns (when the local chicken factory caught fire!). It was literally a baptism of fire and I saw conditions there that I had not seen before (and have never seen since), including Meleney's superficial gangrene (now called necrotizing fasciitis or the flesh-eating bug); polycystic disease of the liver; and acute abdominal distension due to a benign rectal stricture. Mr Hall Drake was a highly experienced and gentle mentor, always patient with my questions and inadequacies. I came to hold him in high regard. He first introduced me to that fascinating condition Crohn's disease and lent me the original monograph on the subject.

Two groups of surgical patients gave me great cause for anxiety: the gall bladders and the prostates. We had a run of postoperative complications with both conditions. In the gallbladder cases, several times in the middle of the night I was called to a patient in severe abdominal pain following the removal of the organ and it turned out that bile (a very irritant substance) had leaked into the peritoneum, a condition called biliary peritonitis. Several patients died. The other problem group were the old men and their prostatectomies. They often bled and had to be transfused. Postoperatively, Mr McFadyean used to stitch the indwelling bladder catheter to the prepuce (foreskin) of the penis to anchor it. One night a patient in a delirious post operative state pulled the inflated balloon back down the urethra which must have been incredibly painful and then pulled half his foreskin off at the same time. When I arrived the stitches and half the foreskin were hanging down and the penis was bleeding profusely. Acting out of pure instinct, I cut across the attached remnant of the foreskin with one stroke of a pair of scissors, put in some local anaesthetic and stitched up the remaining part of the prepuce. Mr McFadyean described it next day as an 'emergency' circumcision. The patient recovered without any further serious problems, his offending member liberally covered with Tincture of Benzoin, a commonly used and strong smelling ointment.

As a result of problems with my poor binocular vision and no depth perception, I was an inadequate surgical assistant. Mr Downie the Surgical Registrar was always complaining about my inadequacies and he was completely justified. I muddled through somehow. I managed eventually to do simple appendectomies, hernias and varicose veins but I was conscious of being on the edge of disaster all the time.

This culminated one night when Mr Downie was on leave and the other Surgical Senior House Officers were off duty. I was the only 'surgeon' in the hospital and I was under strict instructions to telephone Mr Magauran if any emergencies came in. As if to order a case of acute appendicitis arrived! I made the diagnosis and rang Mr Magauran. He said go ahead and operate and Nigel became my assistant! The incision and opening the abdomen were straightforward but I could not find the appendix! After searching for about ten minutes (it seemed like ten hours) we decided to call Mr Magauran who came in from home. He found the appendix in about thirty seconds; it was retrocaecal (behind the caecum) and out it came in short order. 'At least the diagnosis was correct', he

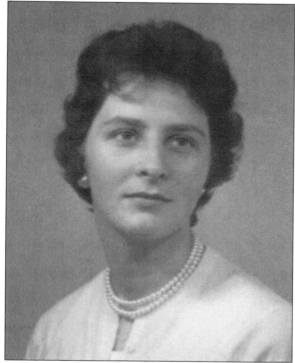

Judith Ann Horrocks (at 21); taken shortly after we met in 1959.

growled in his brusque Glaswegian tones. In retrospect, I was acting beyond my competence and the system should not have allowed it. The same strictures applied to my minor surgical operations, removing lumps and bumps and infantile circumcisions.

As if all this was not exciting and frightening enough, I was about to fall in love again. I went out with one or two of the nurses for a drink, or to the cinema, but there was nothing much to it. Then I met Judith. When I first arrived in Lancaster, she had been away on holiday for a period. One evening I went down to the female surgical ward at about 8 p.m., as was my habit after supper, and there, writing up the report, was Staff Nurse Judith Horrocks SRN. She gave me briefly and competently a run down on all the patients and I never heard a word of it. I was mesmerized! So started a relationship that continues more than forty years on.

We were helped by the fact that I had been moved from the White Hart Hotel, where I had stayed temporarily, to the Lodge, which was a self-contained cottage in the grounds of the Infirmary. This cottage I shared with Roy Atherton who was the surgical Registrar in Orthopaedics. We were able to share passionate trysts in the Lodge far away from the main hospital and the Nurses' Home. On one unforgettable night we were locked in an embrace in my room at the Lodge when Roy Atherton came back. Not knowing we were there he launched into Beethoven's Moonlight Sonata on the piano in the lounge. I never hear this melody without recalling those heady days!

Eventually, after a couple of months, we were sat by the canal one November evening and I asked Judith to marry me. Later on we would agree that we hardly knew each other but after several days' thought Judith agreed. I had to borrow half the money from her for an engagement ring as my munificent salary of £30 per month barely kept body and soul together.

The news of our engagement went round the closed community like a brush fire! Mr Hall Drake met me in the corridor on the following Monday morning and to my surprise said, 'What's this I hear! Congratulations'. He had operated on Judith for acute appendicitis the year before and she had always been one of his favourite staff nurses. I took Judith to Manchester where my father immediately asked whether she was a Roman Catholic! In fact she had been brought up as a Methodist at Keswick in the English Lakes.

I was offered another job in the Casualty Department at the hospital but the time had come to leave Lancaster. I was to go back to Manchester, as Douglas Black's house physician, on M1 Ward at the Royal Infirmary. Judith would do Part One Midwifery at Crumpsall Hospital (where I had been born twenty-five years earlier). I left Surgery with no regrets. I am lost in admiration for those who pursue this arduous vocation but it was not for me. My body and eyes were simply not up to it. I was seeking the more gentlemanly life of the physician with, hopefully, an academic flavour. I had now set sail into the maelstrom of the Professorial Medical Unit at Manchester for six months before the mast. The captain of the ship would be my second giant, Professor Douglas Black, Fellow of the Royal College of Physicians of London.

CHAPTER 11

Manchester Again (1960)

Some fell by laudanum, and some by steel,
And death in ambush lay in every pill.
Sir Samuel Garth
1661-1719
The Dispensary IV 62

O N THE LAST DAY of January 1960 I moved into the doctors' residence at the Manchester Royal Infirmary. Peter Fentem, my immediate predecessor as M1 houseman, waited on my arrival with some anxiety. I would understand his disquiet clearly some six months later when my relief was expected! The next period of half a year would bear close resemblance to a short prison sentence or to a voyage around Cape Horn in a windjammer! I was on call continuously, with only the short respite periods of Thursday evening between 6 p.m. and 10 p.m. and Sunday between lunchtime and 10 p.m. The rest of the time I was at the mercy of the 'bleep' during the day or the telephone in my room during the night. The work was non-stop and relentless. There was no sympathy from our superiors – they had done it; why shouldn't we? As I will point out later working to the point of exhaustion led to frayed tempers and mistakes.

The first thing the new housemen had to do was to parade before the consultants so that they were able to recognize their 'slaves' for the next six months. I say housemen – there was one woman amongst us – she must have felt very isolated. Ninety percent of us were unmarried; to be on the house was a marriage fracturing experience!

After this cattle market was over, I reported to the wards and began the long battle against disease and my superiors. The house physician, being at the bottom of the totem pole, was the butt of all failures and deficiencies, as the Senior Registrar 'kicked' the Senior House Officer and they both castigated me. Everything had to be in apple pie order for the

Professor's Ward Round where I had to present the clinical cases and face a barrage of criticism on diagnosis, treatment and management.

One particular thorn in my flesh was Geoffrey Berlyne! He was the finest medical graduate at Manchester for a decade and had an encyclopaedic knowledge of Medicine. He criticized all my diagnoses! To some degree Douglas Black and Bill Stanbury took pity on me at the post-ward round discussions and shielded me somewhat. After about a month of this harassment I decided to take Geoffrey on and with my Oxford background in physiology and biochemistry began to argue with him. I eventually won a bout by telling him that a differential diagnosis of periodic hypokalaemic paralysis (in China) was Pa Ping or chronic barium poisoning! Reluctantly we were to develop a grudging respect for each other. He is now a distinguished Professor of Renal Medicine in New York.

These discussions in the departmental library could become very heated and, on one occasion, after Professor Black had gone away, Bill Stanbury called us all back and gave the assembled group a real 'telling off' for being rude to the Head of Department. We had hardly noticed! I came to appreciate the Professor's knowledge of the electrolytes and kidney disease and even more his dry wit and common sense. He never trumpeted his knowledge but he had an uncanny knack of getting to the heart of the matter. He could also, with wry humour, keep Dr Berlyne in check! I decided that I would like to work with (and for) him if the opportunity presented itself.

The clinical pounding continued relentlessly. I was clerking patients at midnight and doing pleural aspirations at 4 o'clock in the morning. My diagnostic skill improved in leaps and bounds. In one week, I remember admitting the following: Klinefelter's syndrome with acute pancreatitis; cerebellar abscess due to chronic suppurative middle ear disease; spontaneous haemothorax; and chronic renal failure with malignant hypertension.

I saw Judith rarely and when I went home to Tweedale, on a Sunday afternoon, I would sleep in the armchair for several hours and then drag myself back to the Infirmary. Mother thought my treatment inhumane and it brought back all her fears about rheumatic fever! She said that she would write and complain to Professor Black but I dissuaded her from doing so!

The only think that kept me going was the fixation that this ordeal had a finite end (31 July 1960) and I marked the days off, as we moved towards this Nirvana. Due to fatigue I began to make mistakes, although fortunately none were crucial. I now had to consider what to do at the beginning of August. The normal progression for the M1 house physician was to become a Resident Clinical Pathologist for a year. This involved cross-matching blood and doing simple biochemical tests at night. I decided in my usual arrogant way that I did not want to be a laboratory technician so I would not apply. I did put myself forward for a Senior House Officer Post in Medicine and was turned down like the proverbial bedspread! I then became irritated. I would have to move away from Manchester to find a Senior House Officer post that hopefully would give me some free time to read for the Membership.

At this point, the dreaded National Service loomed its ugly head! As housemen we were exempt from Service but once this period was over we were liable to be called up. I was summoned for a medical examination at premises in Knott Mill, Manchester.

I gave this problem considerable thought. Should I go in the Army Medical Corps? The idea did not appeal at all as I thought I would end up inspecting conscripts with athlete's foot at Catterick Camp in Yorkshire! It was time to play the rheumatic card! I filled the proforma out with great relish and ended with the statement, 'now suffering from rheumatic mitral incompetence'. I also took the precaution of doing ten toe-touching exercises before the examining doctor came to my cubicle, the classic method of making a cardiac murmur louder. 'Well you certainly have a murmur,' he said. 'You'll have to go and see a cardiac Specialist.'

Two weeks later, I appeared (in white coat) before Dr Morgan Jones, consultant cardiologist at the Royal Infirmary, who knew me well. He listened carefully and said, 'Well you have certainly got a mitral murmur. Do you want to go in the Service?' I replied like a shot from a gun, 'No, I want to get married and do the MRCP.' I think it was in that order! He grunted and went off. The next week my Army Medical card came through; I had been graded C3 (unfit for Service). That was that!

I began to look for a post outside Manchester and to prepare for my marriage to Judith. As the British Medical Journal came in, week by week, I turned immediately to the back pages where the job advertisements were placed. I wanted a non-resident house officer post, where I would have

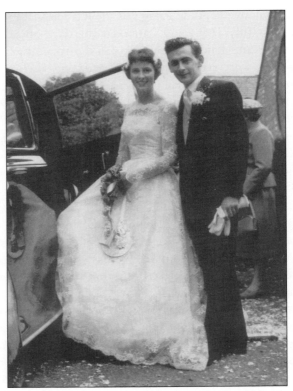

Southey St Methodist Church, Keswick, Cumberland
on the 27th of August 1960.

time to read for the Membership. Eventually a post came up, in South
Wales, with the Medical Research Council Pneumoconiosis Research
Unit at Llandough Hospital. I rang up the director of the Unit, Dr John
Gilson, and he encouraged me to apply. I spoke to Douglas Black who
said he would support me and off I went to Cardiff to be interviewed by
Drs Gilson, McKerrow and Cotes. I found out later that the post was
regarded as a 'backwater' and they had only had two applicants. I was
offered the post and accepted it with the proviso that I could have two
weeks off in August to get married!

The rest of the time at Manchester passed quickly. The clinical load
eased slightly as the summer months came in. I sought a departing
interview with Douglas Black and, emboldened by my imminent

separation from the Royal Infirmary told him that I was absolutely exhausted by my 130 hours a week on call (with only one week's holiday). He agreed that they should attempt to share house physicians with Haematology in the near future to ease the workload. He advised me to get the Membership as soon as I could and, with his usual quizzical sense of humour, also to tone down my knowledge of neurology as it might be too much for the average examiner who was not a neurologist! I said that I hoped I would be able to do some research on the kidney with him in the future at some stage. He said he would welcome the idea and I departed from the presence of my second giant. I was indeed to work on the kidney but sadly never with Douglas Black.

In the afternoon, my successor as M1 house physician arrived and I greeted him with the joy shown in Wild West films for the advent of the Seventh Cavalry! I showed him the assembled patients and went off to the Mess Party. The Resident Medical Officer, Kim Medley, looked gloomy. 'I now have to get used to a whole new batch of housemen who are just qualified and wet behind the ears,' he said plaintively! So the unceasing round and rhythm of the teaching hospital had moved on its inexorable way and the next group of trusting innocents had arrived.

I was too tired to drink much beer and at about ten o'clock Nigel drove me home to Blackley. I was filled with a mixture of emotions: joy at escaping the treadmill of the house physician's lot, and ineffable sadness that the parting of the ways with Nigel had come. We had been blood brothers for seven years and had, together, come through all that the medical course and the pre-registration year could throw at us. He was to stay in Manchester and became a very distinguished surgeon there. I was off to Welsh Wales where, unknown to me, my third giant was waiting!

CHAPTER 12

Cardiff and Archie Cochrane (1960-1961)

The Price of Coal is Men's Lives.
Anonymous

The MRC Pneumoconiosis Research Unit was set at the end of a long corridor at Llandough Hospital, in its own block, which comprised offices, laboratories, a library and a dedicated X-ray department. Across the corridor was a sixteen-bedded clinical ward where the miners (and others) with industrial lung disease were admitted. Miners were taken in from all over the Welsh coalfield for many sorts of studies, principally X-ray progression, physiology and so on. One of my first sad duties was to attend a post-mortem on one of the colliers where, I was informed, one lung went to the National Coal Board and one to the Miner's Union so that any later dispute about compensation could be resolved!

As soon as I became acquainted with the miners my regard for their courage and stoicism rose in leaps and bounds. Pneumoconiosis sometimes proceeds to a particularly nasty complication called progressive massive fibrosis in which large sections of lung are destroyed by fibrosis and cavitation. Acute melanoptysis (coughing coal) or even haemoptysis (coughing blood) can occur. On one occasion one of the miners literally drowned in his own blood as a result of massive haemoptysis, the most distressing death I have ever witnessed. We administered large doses of morphine. As a result his agony was not prolonged. He was in any case unfit for surgery as his overall lung function was so poor.

Occasionally, I went out with the Unit social worker into the pit villages of the Big and Little Rhondda valleys to see disabled miners in their own homes. My memories of these visits are of a succession of cheerful wiry men, in bed downstairs, slowly coughing up the whole of their lungs and saying, 'It's the dust you see', and their indomitable wives giving us tea and cake afterwards. Within a few months, another flag

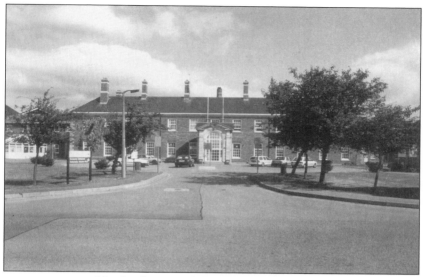

Llandough Hospital near Cardiff, South Wales.

would disappear from the large-scale map of the valleys in the General Office, signalling yet another death to be added to the gloomy statistics.

I was asked by the Unit Director, Dr John Gilson, to work with Dr John Cotes on the physiological testing of miners with dust disease. This involved exercising them on the treadmill and taking samples of arterial and venous blood for analysis of oxygen and carbon dioxide tensions (and oxyhaemoglobin saturations). I was one of the people deputed to use the Van Slyke apparatus to measure these variables. This machine was the handiwork of the devil, combining a maximum of tedium with a maximum of danger! It was very easy to slop mercury over and not all of it was caught by the traps.

In an outburst of my know-all attitudes, I suggested to the Unit chemist that he ought to analyse the mercury concentration of the atmosphere in the gas analysis laboratory. To my satisfaction, and the consternation of the director of the Unit, the atmospheric concentration of mercury came back way over the upper limit permitted! The laboratory was closed for several weeks and the floorboards had to be ripped out. Quicksilver gets everywhere! It would have been very embarrassing if a member of an MRC Unit dedicated to industrial health had gone down with chronic mercurial poisoning! I kept a low profile for a few weeks as I had stopped the work of the laboratory. Nevertheless my first scientific paper came out on the basis of a comparison of gas analysis methods and I felt ten feet high. It was what we would now call a 'pot boiler'!

At this time it was decided that the acute effect of coal dust inhalation should be measured on normal volunteers. A large tent was erected, controlled coal dust aerosols were manufactured and we sat in these tents for eight hours a day. Lung function was measured before and afterwards and then we went to the shower. Essentially the results were negative but it represented my first experience as a normal volunteer. I was to continue volunteering for such activities until I was nearly 50 years old, when, as will be seen later, I could no longer be regarded as 'normal'.

At about this time we had a 'visit' by the Secretary of the Medical Research Council, Sir Harold Himsworth. I write 'visit' as a euphemism, as it amounted to a three-day inspection in which members of the Unit had to present their work. The level of anxiety generated was considerable but I felt strangely detached as I had no intention of staying at the Unit indefinitely. Sir Harold, who was one of the Barons of Medicine, made a few non-committal remarks at the dinner that was held in his honour and went back to London. It would have been politically inexpedient to close the Unit at that stage and it went on for a number of years until the mine closure programme began to bite.

One day, I was standing in the corridor when a wiry small man with blondy-red hair came along and noticed me squinting at the notice board with my myopic gaze. He said immediately, 'I'm Archie Cochrane and you need an eye test. I'll get you to see Mr Graham, who is a friend of mine, at the Cardiff Royal Infirmary'. This was the start of my friendship with Archie Cochrane who was in charge of the Epidemiology Research Group. True to his word, an appointment to see Mr Graham followed shortly and off I went.

Mr Graham discovered that my right eye had been more seriously affected by the flying stone in childhood than I had imagined. It was amblyopic and there was also a scar on the retina caused by a contra-coup injury. *Pro tanto quid retribuamus!* So shall we be rewarded! However, correcting the myopia of seven dioptres in the left eye improved my vision enormously and I have worn spectacles since for every waking hour.

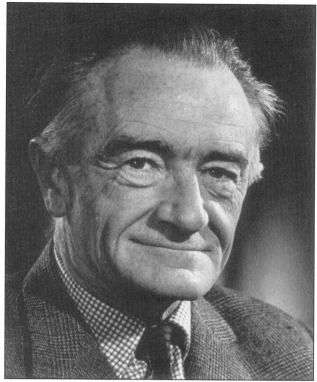

Archibald Leman Cochrane FRCP (1909-1988). Known universally as 'Archie'.

I thanked Archie profusely and from then on Judith and I were regular visitors at his home at Rhoos. Archie Cochrane was very different from any senior doctor that I had encountered up to that time. He was the exact opposite to the 'freemasons' that I shall describe in the next chapter, in that he was antiauthoritarian in most respects and believed very strongly in shining the light of reason into many of the dark crevices of medical knowledge. Allied to this he had no sense of rank and insisted that I call him Archie and he would call me Mike. To this refreshing sense of informality was added a self-deprecating ironic humour. The medical profession found him very difficult to deal with over the years as one by one he attacked their sacred shibboleths!

I told him that I was the son of a shop worker. Further back I was also the grandson of a toffee boiler from Manchester and a docker from

Liverpool, and it would probably be 'Clogs to Clogs in three generations'. This quotation pleased him immensely and he proceeded to relay this quip to the assembling dinner guests. I noted that the farmhouse had a swimming pool, which was unusual for those days. Taken together with one or two fine ornaments, several pieces of sculpture and a fine Chinese ivory chess set, it struck me forcibly that Archie must be a man of independent means.

The next time we met I asked him whether he was a relative of the Cochrane who founded the Chilean Navy (or the 'sea wolf' as Napoleon had called him). Archie did not answer directly. I think, in some moods, he liked to think he was in an illegitimate line from the famous admiral and the Earls of Dundonald. In fact he was the son (and grandson) of wealthy textile manufacturers in Galashiels in the Scottish Borders. His father was killed at Gaza in Palestine in the First World War.

I used to chide him gently that he was rich enough to be a Communist! Later on in life, he would use some of his own capital to fund a Trust for Research in Epidemiology and Public Health. As we got to know each other better, he told me unreservedly about his experiences in the 1930s. Educated at Uppingham and Christ's College Cambridge he had a distinguished undergraduate career taking first class honours. He did not enjoy clinical medicine or laboratory research into tissue culture. At one stage after floating round Europe with his psychotherapist he joined the International Brigade and fought in Spain for a year although he was never a signed up member of the Communist Party. Later he joined the British Army and was taken prisoner of war in Crete in 1941. His reminiscences of the prisoner of war camp were like something out of the *Boy's Own Paper* and, with my strong sense of history, I found them compelling. I particularly liked the stories of his negotiations with the camp commandants, which occurred in such fluent Hochdeutsch (High German), that the Nazis thought he was an aristocrat; which in a way he was!

He tried to persuade me to become an epidemiologist and give up all this nonsense of clinical medicine. He called me a 'phenomenologist' and said that my trouble was that I wanted to do good straight away and was not prepared to wait to do more good in the long term. He was right, of course, but I could not be persuaded.

Occasionally, he would have a group of doctors from behind the Iron Curtain come to visit him as he was thought to be vaguely sympathetic to their views. This was to witness Archie at his best conversing in fluent German, dropping occasionally into French, Italian or Serbo-Croat! Once with a group of Czechs he was able to elicit the fact that they would throw out the Communists (and Russians) tomorrow, if they were able; all this eight years before the 1968 uprising.

Archie's work on pneumoconiosis, chest disease, coronary artery disease and many other disorders became so well known that he came to be in demand to speak at national meetings and international conferences. He did not enjoy flying, claiming that the airlines always lost his baggage (which was partially true) and that he was always ill for a fortnight after he got back with peculiar pains in the abdomen and limbs together with insomnia! We always kidded him that it was a hysterical reaction to flying but in turned out some years later that he had been in the habit of taking barbiturate to help him sleep on long flights (or in foreign hotels) and this would provoke an attack of the rare disease porphyria! Archie then took great (and perverse) pleasure in investigating one hundred and fifty of his relatives for this uncommon and perplexing inherited disease.

The time in Cardiff passed by at the speed of an express train. In the evenings, I practised writing old Membership papers under examination conditions (three hours of non-stop effort). I also read the *Quarterly Journal of Medicine* (the examiners' club journal), which together with the editorials in the *Lancet* and the *British Medical Journal*, became a potential source of written and oral questions for the forthcoming examination.

The day came in April 1961 to report at Queen's Square in London for the written examination of the Membership of the Royal College of Physicians. When I reached Queen's Square I was taken aback! There were 370 candidates packed into two great Halls. Then the practice I had undertaken kicked in and the machine took over. Meningitis; acute renal failure; hypoglycaemic drugs; the juggernaut moved on.

The critical part of the examination were the long and short clinical cases. For these, I had to attend the Royal Free Hospital and face Lee Landor (long case) and Sheila Sherlock and Stokes (short cases). This was not only a test of knowledge and clinical skill but a test of nerve. The long case went well but then I had to face Sheila Sherlock, who had already established a reputation as something of a spitfire. She showed me a man with a huge abdomen, enlarged liver and ascites. I listened to the bowel sounds and said as confidently as I could 'The high pitched bowel sounds of subacute obstruction'. She did not reply but pointed to the abdomen – there were the waves of visible peristalsis which confirmed my diagnosis. 'Large bowel or small bowel' she barked. 'More likely to be large bowel,' I said. 'Good' she said and passed me onto Dr Stokes who, seeing I was carrying my Kieler ophthalmoscope said 'Have a look at these two patients' fundi.'

The first one was straightforward hypertensive retinopathy with haemorrhages; exudates and papilloedema. The second was much more testing; there was optic atrophy on one side and papilloedema on the other. I reported the findings to him and I realized it was a rarum avis or rare bird (as we called it). 'What do you think might cause it?' he said. I thought for an instant; I must go for it and replied 'Foster/Kennedy syndrome – probable tumour in the frontal lobe.' I had hardly finished speaking when the bell went to signal the end of the session and off I went.

I was then summoned to the next stage of the steeplechase, the so-called Pathology Viva, where I answered questions on gout, autoimmune disease, subarachnoid haemorrhage and Sturge-Weber's syndrome. Then came the letter to attend the final viva at the College's Headquarters in Pall Mall. The final viva had legendary, semimythical, status. Everybody knew a Dr X from the Middlesex Hospital, who failed it three times before eventually succeeding; or a Dr Y of the London Hospital who had also failed the test after being asked unanswerable questions about amoebic dysentery and Chaga's disease (South American trypano-somiasis)!

I entered the room to see Sir Robert Platt the President lowering over me from the end of the table, with the Censors on either side. 'Sit down please; good.' I did not know whether this was a comment on my sitting down or my performance. 'I have just one question.' There seemed to be an interminable pause and my heart raced. 'Many people try the French translation in the paper but very few attempt the German. Where did you learn your German?' I replied 'At the Manchester Grammar School, and I have kept it going to a degree ever since.' A slight smile passed across his face as he had been Professor of Medicine at Manchester (before Douglas Black). I gave thanks for Billy Hulme and his tyrannical teaching, seized the white envelope (which meant a pass), and left the room as swiftly as I could manage. I wrote a cheque for thirty guineas which was, in one way, the cheapest life insurance that could be bought. I had passed the Membership Examination of the Royal College of Physicians of London at the first attempt!

I could barely keep still on the train back to Cardiff and embraced Judith with fervour when I arrived home. Of the 370 hardy souls who had started out on the examination, only 35 had passed, a failure rate of about 90%. Donald Acheson (and others) at around that time criticized the examination comprehensively, saying with justification that any test that failed 90% of the candidates was arbitrary and unfair. The examination was extensively reorganized and is now a much better assessment with an overall pass rate of some 30 to 40%.

Archie Cochrane was awarded the MRCP (honoris causa) at the same ceremony at which I received my certificate. I told him, as we travelled up on the train from Cardiff together, that here was he getting in by the back door and I had had to drive myself for two years to gain the elusive diploma! I marvel now at my effrontery! He took it all in good part saying that the Establishment, against which he had fought for so long, was finally taking him in but he would always feel (and behave) like an outsider. He encouraged me to go on asking questions (and criticizing those in authority) even though it would prove at times to be a dangerous strategy.

When I left Cardiff we kept in touch down the years. He kindly sent me a signed copy of his Rock Carling Lecture 'Effectiveness and Efficiency' which was to prove so influential in many ways over the decades. This copy now rests in the Library of the Royal College of Physicians at Edinburgh. As I write in the new Millennium, Cochrane centres are springing up all over the civilized world. I think Archie would have derived a great deal of wry amusement from the fact that what he regarded as Common Sense has now become an industry!

I was sorry to leave Cardiff, the Unit and Archie. It had been a very happy time for Judith and me as a newly married couple. Archie would have both a short term and long term influence on my career. In the short term he would have some influence on my appointment with Sir George Pickering, as he had been working with Sir George in the studies on the epidemiology of essential hypertension in South Wales which led to the famous Platt versus Pickering controversy.

It was the evidence from South Wales that established beyond peradventure that the arterial blood pressure was normally distributed in the population. The controversy between the two great Barons went on for so long in the columns of the medical journals that it spawned its own humour and the waggish remark that 'I'll stop bickering with Pickering and have a bat at Platt!'

In the long term, I would value Archie's experience of life and his outlook on research (and the medical profession). I also took to heart his advice not to take matters (or yourself) too seriously and to try to remember, as Robert Burns had put it so well, 'The rank is but the guinea's stamp. The man's the gowd for a'that.'

I decided to explore the possibility of returning to mainstream medicine in general and to Oxford University in particular. Armed with the MRCP diploma, and a sense of my own importance, I wrote to Professor Leslie Witts, the Nuffield Professor of Medicine at the Radcliffe Infirmary, to explore the possibility of doing research in haematology (pernicious anaemia was speaking again!). Unfortunately, he had no vacancies at that time but intimated that he had heard that there might be a junior post coming up in the Regius Professor of Medicine's department at the same hospital (Head, Sir George Pickering FRCP, FRS). Sure enough, within a few weeks, the post of Junior Lecturer in Medicine in Sir George's department was advertised in the medical press and I decided to apply. Before I relate what was to happen next, I must make a short digression into the state of academic medicine in Britain in the 1960s, as it was to play an integral part in my chequered progress over the next ten years.

CHAPTER 13

The Barons and Freemasons of Medicine

For Brutus is an honourable man:
So are they all, all honourable men.
Julius Caesar III ii 88

IN THE 1960s, Medicine was ruled by a series of barons who were Professors and Heads of Departments. They included for example, Pickering (Oxford); McMichael (The Hammersmith Hospital); Wilson (the London Hospital); Himsworth followed by Rosenheim (University College Hospital); Davidson (Edinburgh); Wayne (Glasgow); Stuart-Harris (Sheffield); Sharpey-Schäfer (St Thomas' Hospital); Platt followed by Black (Manchester); and Cohen (Liverpool). In general there were no women until Sheila Sherlock broke the mould by her appointment at the Royal Free Hospital; very few Jews apart from those at University College Hospital (UCH which was known as Jew CH); and certainly no one from the Indian subcontinent.

The barons influenced anything and everything. Sometimes their rule was benign, sometimes not so. They had a major effect on appointments to both University and NHS posts; and on the distribution of research grants and Merit (or Distinction awards). They were known colloquially to those of us in the junior ranks as Big Wheels and it was essential if you were to make progress in academic (and indeed NHS) Medicine that you worked for a spell with one of these major movers and shakers.

This led in general to two conflicting attitudes which were held by the staff of their departments: the first being fear leading to sycophancy and the second to an occasional rebellion. The second attitude could lead to the setting up of a splinter group which would compete fiercely with its 'mother' department. As a consequence scientific meetings could be the scenes of vitriolic exchanges where one group would try to put another down.

The Barons could influence an individual's career both for good or bad. This had several undesirable effects. For example, a mediocre physician could progress to a Chair having received continuous strong support from his Baron, whereas somebody who had caused 'trouble' might find themselves posted to a consultant post in Slagtown, Scunsby or Grimville in the frozen North (the equivalent of exile in Siberia)! An even more radical solution would result in certain individuals going down the Brain Drain to the Old Colonies of America, Australia and New Zealand! It is rumoured that when one of the Barons was asked about the Brain Drain, which was a serious problem in the 1960s, he replied succinctly, 'Some come; some go; who cares?' There would always be willing volunteers to take the place of the casualties.

There was always the possibility of moving, if circumstances decreed, into a so-called 'lesser' unattractive speciality, for example Radiology, Psychiatry, Geriatrics or even, perish the thought, Laboratory Medicine!

The other serious problem that Medicine had in the 1960s was what I will call 'freemasonry'. Joining the profession was akin to entering a secret society. There was an unspoken oath of secrecy to cover up mistakes and keep them away from patients and their relatives, and in particular the Medical Defence Unions together with the General Medical Council. If an 'accident' occurred, the doctor who had committed the error would be dealt with harshly by his senior colleagues. They would then lie through their back teeth to the patient/and or their relatives. This course of action was helped by the fact that the public was in general much less well-informed than it is today. Whistle-blowers were virtually unknown and had no protection.

What is the situation forty years on? First, as to the Barons and the Baronies. The number of departments and Chairs must have tripled over the intervening period and, as a consequence, the effect that one single Professor can have has been very much diluted. Second, academic medicine is no longer an attractive career and there is a major recruitment crisis. Third, a good deal of research money comes not from the Universities (or the Medical Research Council) but from the Wellcome Trust and in particular the pharmaceutical industry. These purse string holders have different priorities.

As to freemasonry, a series of major scandals overtook the profession in the 1990s, including the Bristol Heart Scandal and the Alder Hey Organ

Retention debacle. As a result, all the regulations have changed and we now have accreditation, audit and appraisal of physicians and departments. The secret society is being broken into fragments and not before time. Hopefully the general public will retain its confidence in the medical profession through the recent mayhem but it has been 'a damned close run thing'.

I must now return to my narrative – I had applied for a job with a Big Wheel – Sir George Pickering FRCP. FRS. Regius Professor of Medicine at the University of Oxford. It will be recalled that it was this man whom Eric James had recommended to me in 1953, when I left Manchester Grammar School for Oxford University. In the meantime George Pickering had moved from his chair at St Mary's in London to Oxford, having been appointed by the Queen (hence Regius or Royal).

CHAPTER 14

Into Sir George's Lane
(1961-1969)

'O Let me lead an academicke life'
B. Hall. Virgidem, 1599 IV; 83

Oxford – home of lost causes and
forsaken beliefs, and unpopular names
and impossible loyalties!

Matthew Arnold
Essays in Criticism
First Series. Preface

I ARRIVED AT Oxford Station in April 1961 with mixed feelings. My
three years at Brasenose had not been an unmitigated blessing; hard
unrelenting toil followed by a favourable outcome. This time however I
would have Judith with me, which should make all the difference. I
walked up from the station and the old familiar sites came into view;
Worcester College; the Ashmolean Museum; and then passing the Eagle
and Child public house up the Woodstock Road into the Radcliffe
Infirmary. After finding the right staircase, I ascended to be greeted
immediately by a large sign across the corridor which read, 'Sir George's
Lane'! Of course this was a grandiose claim; during my time in the
department it had to be taken down on one occasion when a national
committee came to inspect us!

I was ushered into the Great Man's presence. He did not rise to greet
me; I later discovered that he had bilateral osteoarthritis of the hips. He
looked at my letter and said, 'Is that right, you obtained First Class
Honours in Physiology?' I answered in the affirmative. At that moment
the phone rang and he uttered an expletive, answered it and told his
secretary he wanted no more calls. He then asked me how Archie
Cochrane was and what he was up to. Without hearing my reply fully he
hobbled to the door and shouted in a loud voice, 'Bill'. Within a moment

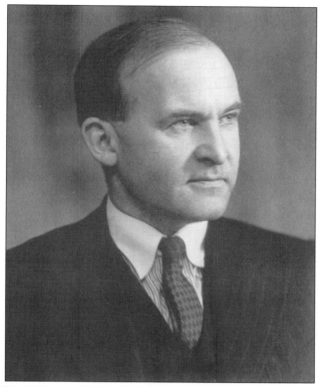

George White Pickering FRCP, FRS (1904-1980). One-time Regius Professor of Medicine at the University of Oxford and later Master of Pembroke College at the same University.

(or two) Bill Brown, his technician, appeared and he grunted, 'Now Bill, show Dr Lee round the department' and then in an aside to me, 'You'll be up for interview next week'. He turned awkwardly on his heels and disappeared into his office. The whole thing must have taken all of three minutes. Bill Brown, who I was to get to know very well later on, showed me round the department and told me something of the research that was taking place there. I walked slowly back to the station reflecting 'Curiouser and Curiouser'. I later learned that this was an absolutely typical interview! One of Sir George's American visitors once described a meeting with the Professor as like trying to 'stand on a grasshopper in a field'.

The next week came the formal interview and I ended up being offered the post for two years. Judith and I moved to Oxford, first to a flat in Rectory Road (off Cowley Road) and then to our first home in the village of Finstock, which was in the country between Witney and Charlbury. Home life was very happy but this was more than could be said for research. I had the naive idea that within three to six months the results would be rolling out and recognition would soon follow. I did not realize that there was another apprenticeship to be served in order to become technically competent. This involved weighing, measuring, titrating, centrifuging and analysing. I was in something of an emotional hangover after the Membership examination and my spirits and energy remained low for some months.

I did not like the project that the Professor had given me, to study the effect of angiotension (a vasopressor polypeptide) on the rabbit kidney. Much to his annoyance, I asked him if I could work with his research student Bill Cook who had just finished his D.Phil (Doctor of Philosophy degree). 'What are you going to try and do?' growled the Regius. Bill replied, 'We would like to estimate renin activity in the plasma'. This was the Holy Grail of work on renal hypertension and Pickering had worked on it himself in the 1930s (with Prinzmetal at University College Hospital). 'You know Stan Peart and his team are working on it at St Mary's?' Reluctantly he agreed to us working together on the project.

I learned a great deal from Bill Cook. He was disorganized and his laboratory was often shambolic. He had nevertheless come up the hard way; en route he had been a GPO Telegraph boy, a laboratory technician, and now had become a Doctor of Philosophy. He had done (or seen done) most techniques in laboratory medicine. He told me straightaway that failure was inevitable, success rare, and Eureka moments came to the fortunate about once in every ten years. He liked to work an unusual schedule from about eleven in the morning to nine at night, punctuated by a session in the Royal Oak public house in the Woodstock Road for two pints of beer (and light refreshments)!

Progress was pitifully slow for the first two years but then we had two strokes of luck. The first was to find that on removing the kidneys in rabbits and hence the source of endogenous renin, the production of its substrate (the substance renin acted on) by the animal's liver, increased four to five-fold. This allowed us to obtain preparations of the substrate that were very pure and very active. The second shaft of fate, which was to produce a Eureka moment, was the discovery that when renin made angiotensin, from its substrate, normally the peptide product would be destroyed rapidly by enzymes (called angiotensinases). By adding the heavy metals, cadmium and mercury, these 'ase' enzymes could be blocked. Meanwhile Lever, Robertson and Tree at St Mary's had published their method which was excellent and clarified many important clinical problems in clinical hypertension. We were way behind! Sir George began to show some concern and asked Bill Cook if I would like to transfer to St Mary's (on the basis if you can't beat them join them)! Judith and I were invited to dinner at Norham Gardens (the Regius' official residence) and he asked her if I was depressed and told her that it was a very tough problem that we were working on.

Within a month of this second conversation, all our problems resolved and we had a workable method, more sensitive than that developed by the St Mary's group in that it could be carried out on five millilitres of venous blood (compared to their 40 millilitres). Sir George was delighted and when Bill Cook told him the news, he held him by both elbows and grinned widely. This was a rare accolade and was known to us all as the 'double elbow grip and mazurka'!

I was able shortly afterwards to submit my Doctor of Philosophy Thesis entitled, 'The Estimation of Renin in Biological Fluids'. This was an education in itself as I had to take the drafts of my chapters to the Regius in Norham Gardens for his amendments and approval. A painful and lengthy process then ensued as he had embarked on a personal crusade on the use of English, epitomized by his address on 'Language the Lost Tool of Learning'! His usual recommendations were the King James version of the Bible and Roget's Thesaurus. I did manage to catch him out on one occasion when he asked had I read Tigerstedt's and Bergman's original description of the discovery of renin in 1898 and I replied absolutely truthfully, 'Yes, in the original German! *Niere und Kreislauf* (the Kidneys and the Circulation)'!

At long last the work was finished and submitted. The internal examiner was Dr Walker who promptly developed hepatitis and as a result delayed, through no fault of his own, the viva voce examination. Stan Peart, the Professor of Medicine at St Mary's (our rivals) would be, as expected, the external examiner. I sweated on the top line for almost six months but finally the long deferred day came. Dr Walker said very little but held the ring. Stan Peart questioned me for about two hours and as he was a giant in the field, I felt as if I was going through the mangle. He asked me finally to criticize the St Mary's method and compare it to ours at Oxford. I tried to be as fair as I could.

At long last he had exhausted his two foolscap pages of questions and said, 'Well done! We'll let you know,' and went off to have lunch at Norham Gardens with the Regius. I knew he was going there because he told me so! There had been some tension between the two great men but it had been resolved. I staggered up the Woodstock Road to the Royal Oak public house and sank two pints of bitter in rapid time. Early in the afternoon I drifted back to the Department, still wearing my academic subfusc, including a white bow tie, which was somewhat incongruous in a clinical laboratory setting! Out popped the Regius from his office. 'How did it go?' This was dissembling, as he would already have had a blow-by-blow account from Stan! I replied, 'Alright, I think. There were several difficult questions'. The Regius harrumphed and disappeared.

In retrospect it had been the hardest task I had ever undertaken because the output (in results) bore no relationship to the amount of work put in. Indeed, on numerous occasions, I had felt like giving up. The examiners had to decide whether the work was 'of sufficient merit that it was worthy of publication'. Indeed, in my case, one important paper had already been published in the *Biochemical Journal*. Their verdict came back in the affirmative; I had succeeded! Sir George congratulated me and I was awarded a full Lectureship in Medicine accompanied by his standard homily on not resting on my laurels but continuing to work hard.

At this stage fortune intervened. A young man in the RAF at Cosford in the Midlands developed very severe hypertension and, to cut a long story short, had his kidney removed which cured his high blood pressure. On examination of the kidney there was an unusual tumour in the upper pole (see Figure). Philip Robertson brought some of the tumour down from the RAF hospital and asked me if it would be possible to analyse it for renin. By this time, Bill Cook had gone to a career post in the Pharmacology Department (as a Lecturer) and I decided to enlist the help of Bill Brown, the Professor's technician.

This was an inspired choice as he was one of the best animal handlers and cannulators of blood vessels I have ever encountered. We would have

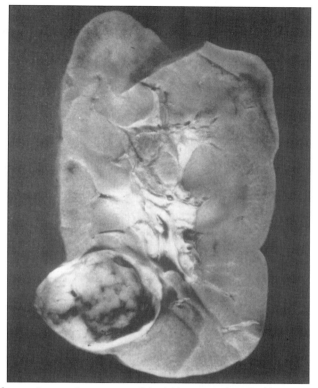

The first renin secreting tumour of the kidney was described by our research group in 1967 in the American Journal of Medicine.

to work on the cat, as human renin acts on cat substrate, but not on that of rat, rabbit or dog. This presented some practical problems as cats are notoriously difficult to anaesthetize and may go fighting mad! Bill had handled them before and proved expert with ethyl chloride and ether.

We measured the blood pressure by a cannula in a main artery and injected a saline extract of the tumour. To our amazement, the blood pressure in the manometer rose and went on rising, looking as though it would never stop! The tumour contained very large amounts of renin. This was another Eureka moment! Over the next few weeks we confirmed these results and this was the first renin-secreting tumour ever to be described. The syndrome is now well known and has been described up to 100 times and is called primary reninism (primary overproduction of renin). The tumour is not only important in itself (as a rare but remediable cause of severe hypertension) but also led to further evaluation of the role of renin in renal artery stenosis (narrowing) and chronic renal failure. Moreover renin would eventually be purified and its chemical structure established from a similar tumour discovered in France. To my surprise, I became well-known in this field, both in North America and on the Continent, and I began to receive offers to go down the 'Brain Drain'. The pressure of work in the mad dash to the Doctor of Philosophy followed by the studies on the renin-secreting tumour had been considerable but it was now important to refresh my clinical skills and to do some teaching. Bill Cranston who had been First Assistant to the Regius had gone to St Thomas's Hospital as Professor of Medicine and Tony Mitchell became First Assistant (Senior Lecturer). He wanted a rest from supervising the clinical wards so I took over for a period of six months. I found this very exciting as I could exercise my diagnostic skills without the drudgery of all the routine work. A number of interesting diagnostic problems turned up including Creutzfeld Jacob disease, Alport's syndrome (hereditary nephritis with deafness) and an insulin-secreting tumour of the pancreas. I was picking it up again and bearing out our visiting Professor, Robert Loeb's dictum, that it was like 'riding a bicycle; you never forget how although you might be a bit wobbly on first getting back on'.

My tour de force came one day in outpatients. A middle-aged man presented with the unusual complaint that a large amount of clear fluid was coming down his nose every day! Rejecting my initial reaction, that this was a major mental delusion, I asked him to collect some. Sure enough he came back with a container holding some twenty to thirty millilitres. I tested the fluid for glucose and to my surprise and delight it was positive! Here was a case of cerebrospinal fluid leaking from the brain down into the nose and out. I referred him to Mr Macbeth the Consultant Ear Nose and Throat surgeon, who together with the neurosurgeons removed an osteoma (benign tumour of bone) from his frontal sinus which had burrowed both into the brain above and the nose below.

Macbeth wrote to Sir George congratulating him on the diagnosis with a copy to M. Radcliffe Lee. I was summoned to the Professor's presence and asked who M. Radcliffe Lee of the Radcliffe Infirmary was. I replied that Radcliffe was my middle name and that in order not to be confused with Grant de Jersey Lee who was a consultant cardiologist at our hospital, I signed myself as Radcliffe Lee. I don't think the Regius was too impressed by my grandiose idea but he could not really fault the logic of my argument!

I was also responsible for the teaching on our Unit but this proved to be an easy task. There were only thirty clinical students a year in Osler House at that time and at any one period there would only be two or three on our Unit. This meant that they could have one-to-one tutorial and bedside teaching. Sir George tried always to attain a 100% pass rate for these students and this was usually achieved in Medicine and Surgery. The Professor of Obstetrics, Chassar Moir sometimes insisted on failing the occasional student in his subject *'pour encourager les autres'*. This led to a few pitched battles in the Examiner's meetings between the two distinguished Professors. I was to reflect later how privileged these Oxford students were, when compared with academic years of 120 individuals (at Leeds) and then 180 (at Edinburgh).

As I entered 1967, I was married with two children, both born in the Radcliffe, and qualified MA; D.Phil (Oxon); MRCP (London); PSP (published several papers). The next qualification required in those competitive days was BTA (Been to America). I therefore applied for a British Heart Foundation Travelling Fellowship. The questions loomed – if it was awarded where should I go and what would I do when I got there?

As I have pointed out earlier, the way we detected renin (and its products angiotensin I and angiotensin II) was to inject these substances into a rat, cat or dog and measure the rise in blood pressure (the so-called bioassay). These bioassays were long, tedious, and expensive. In order to make faster progress we needed a chemical assay that could in the end be largely automated. The answer lay in a technique that used antibodies and isotopically labelled proteins or peptides (the so-called immunoassay). I had to learn how to carry out the technique of immunoassay and then apply the technique to renin (or angiotensin).

There were only two laboratories in the world in the late 1960s where these techniques were being carried out: in the Bronx in New York (Yalow and Berson on insulin) and at the National Institutes of Health in Bethesda, Maryland (Potts and Auerbach on parathyroid hormone). I did not fancy moving my family and myself to the Bronx! Accordingly, I wrote to Dr John Potts, Jr at Bethesda, Maryland and asked if he could accommodate me for a year in his laboratory.

The reply came back in the positive! All I had to do now was to fund myself (and family) to go to Bethesda on the outskirts of Washington (District of Columbia). I went to the interview in London at the British Heart Foundation and was asked by Professor McMichael why I wanted to work on parathyroid hormone, when so far all my work had been on renin and angiotensin. I explained patiently the difficulties of the bioassay and the emerging promise of the technique of immunoassay. The committee grasped the point immediately and completely and I was awarded the Travelling Fellowship. The other advantage was that it was at American rates of pay ($18,000; a small fortune in British terms) together with travelling expenses. I would have some money for the first time in my professional life!

Preparations continued hot foot. Through the kindness of an American friend Philip Gorden, I rented a house in Bethesda. I also bought an Austin 1100 which I exported free of Purchase Tax to the United States. I bade farewell to the Regius who very kindly agreed to extend my Lectureship for a year when I returned to Oxford. I left him with conflicting feelings. I had had a wonderful time in the Regius Professor's department at Oxford, after a very shaky start, and had obtained a postgraduate degree. Our work had made some impact on the research world of renin and hypertension. However, I now felt that I needed to have my own research group where I would not, all the time, be looking over my shoulder at Sir George. Already there had been some irritations over lectures; him borrowing my slides and future lines of research. I wanted to be my own man and go my own way for better or worse!

For the time being these long-term problems were subsumed in the excitement of the Great American dream. As the title of Jack Jones' novel has it; 'It was off to Philadelphia in the Morning' or at least off to Bethesda, Maryland!

CHAPTER 15

An American Frenzy
(1967-1968)

The Land of the Free and the Home of the Brave
American National Anthem

A S WE ENTERED the dock area of Southampton, we could see the three great funnels of the *Queen Mary* looming over the embarkation shed. Before we could load the Austin 1100, it had to be steam-cleaned underneath to prevent the possibility of importing potato eelworm into the United States! At last, when boarding was allowed, Judith and I, together with the children, descended the companionway and found our four-berth cabin in one of the lower decks. The ship was like a great city and we spent several hours exploring. She departed next morning, via Cherbourg, for New York. As it was the last east-to-west voyage, a band played her away; and with a great blast on the siren she slipped slowly away into the Solent. There were two memorable moments in the five-day voyage: the first was passing the *Queen Elizabeth* in mid Atlantic at a range of about two miles. Both great liners sounded their hooters. The second was hearing by shore-to-ship telephone of the launch at Glasgow of the *Queen Elizabeth II* which was celebrated by a champagne reception.

After five days' sailing, early one morning we passed closely under the Verrazano Narrows bridge and then hard by the Statue of Liberty. We then came slowly into dock under the Manhattan skyline. It was a poignant moment as the *Mary*, in honour of her long service, was greeted by the New York fireboats throwing plumes of water into the air.

We then had a long anticlimactic wait until our car was unloaded and we had passed through Customs, before we could set off for Washington DC down the New Jersey turnpike. The 400 miles to the capital was a hair-raising experience, driving, for the first time, on the wrong side of the road and being pursued by huge trucks belching fumes from their smokestacks. Fortunately they gave our peculiar automobile, the tiny

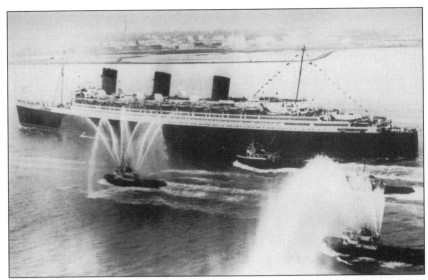

The RMS Queen Mary *leaves Southampton for New York in September 1967 on her last east to west voyage. Note the flags flying and the salute from the fire tugs.*

1100, a wide berth, sounding their klaxons as they went by us as if to say, 'what the hell is this?' After an overnight stay in a motel near the Susquehanna Bridge in Delaware, we rolled into Bethesda, Maryland in mid afternoon on a beautiful day with the temperature in the mid-70s.

Without too much difficulty we found Wessling Lane and the house number 5114 that was to be our home for the next year. Why do the Americans have such peculiar street numbers, the children asked? Bethesda was a leafy suburb of Washington DC but nominally in Maryland, not in the city. The weather was to be beautiful for the next six weeks and then the trees turned into a riot of colour as the Fall came. For the first period we behaved like tourists and visited the Senate on Capital Hill, the Washington memorial, the Museums, Arlington military cemetery and the Great Falls of the Potomac. Later on we would go as far as George Washington's home and the Shenandoah Valley. This was more like a holiday than work!

After a few days I went down to the Clinical Centre of the National Institutes of Health to meet my new leader John Potts. The size of the Centre was overwhelming; at one time it was said to be the largest brick

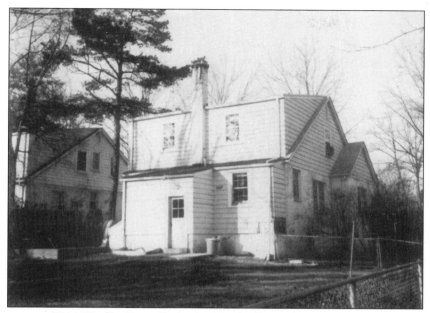

5114 Wessling Lane, Bethesda, Maryland. Our home in America.

building in the world. Here the Federal Government spent enormous amounts of money on medical research. There were countless workers, the number swollen by people avoiding the Vietnam war by joining the Public Health Service.

John Potts was a hard driving pleasant East Coast investigator. He worked both himself and his team relentlessly. He spoke with suppressed excitement in his voice. 'I will call you Mike. You are going to work with Len Deftos. This is a hot ticket!' It turned out that the group had largely switched the focus of their work from parathyroid hormone to thyrocalcitonin; a polypeptide synthesized and stored in the parafollicular cells (C cells) of the thyroid gland. This hormone, on release into the circulation, lowered the blood calcium concentration.

Potts was excited because his group had now isolated a very pure preparation of calcitonin from pig thyroid glands and they were therefore in a powerful position in the race to determine its peptide structure. This would be done by breaking up the aminoacid building blocks of the peptide and establishing the exact sequence of these groups. I was to join

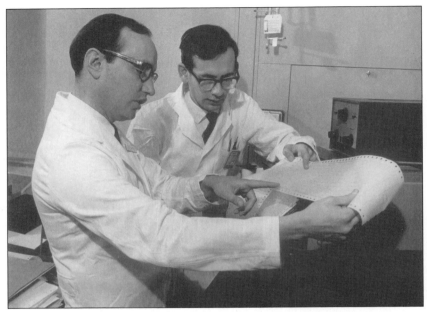

Leonard Deftos (on the left) and I study a print-out of I^{131} – labelled thyrocalcitonin in the laboratory at the National Institutes of Health.

Len Deftos in trying to raise an antibody to the peptide by injecting porcine calcitonin into guinea pigs who were also given Freund's adjuvant (basically mashed up dead tubercle bacilli!) to stimulate their immune systems. The work started immediately and for a few months nothing developed at all. Meanwhile, two other events occurred, each of which was to have a long-term significance in the next few years. The first was that I was summoned by the Public Health Service for a 'medical'. This was the usual routine for all new employees. The physician who examined me noted my cardiac murmur, said I was otherwise fit, and did a standard Mantoux test for tuberculosis. This came up like an egg; in other words I had recently been exposed to tuberculosis and might be incubating the disease. Chest X-ray and laryngeal swabs (for the tuberculosis bacillus) proved negative but he advised me to take six months isoniazid, an antibiotic active against this organism, which I said I would think about, but never got around to. Once again my 'I know best' attitude would prove costly two years later!

At about the same time, I received word from Oxford that my mentor, Sir George Pickering, was to retire and take up the Mastership of Pembroke College at the University. He had become increasingly disabled by osteoarthritis of both hips and the workload of the Regius Professorship had become excessive. The Mastership of Pembroke also had the advantage that it could be held until the age of seventy years. This was a blow and meant that any return to Oxford that I might make at the end of 1968, would certainly only be for a short period, as an incoming Professor would be very unlikely to be interested in essential and renal hypertension.

Up till January, nothing of any excitement happened in Potts' laboratory. I remember the winter months only for very heavy snowfalls and an outbreak of streptococcal pharyngitis in Judith and the children (confirmed by culture of throat swabs at the Clinical Centre). Everybody was treated with penicillin to avoid ping-pong infections.

Then, as February moved into March, everything began to happen at once and the annus mirabilis began! First the structure group put together the final pieces of the porcine calcitonin molecule and confirmed that it was correct. Then one of the guinea pigs produced a fine antibody to thyrocalcitonin and in what seemed like a blink of an eye, Deftos and I were able to measure calcitonin in blood. This was another Eureka moment! These discoveries provoked a frenzy of activity. We worked, for a period of three months, seven days a week and eight hours a day! Wives and families began to complain but we had to beat the opposition to the punch. In the last week of May, John Potts released the news simultaneously to the *Washington Post* and the *New York Times*. There was also a spread in the *NIH Record* of May 28th. We became famous for 24-hours!

Pharmaceutical companies beat a path to Potts' door and soon calcitonin was a commercial proposition. Indeed various preparations of porcine, salmon and other calcitonins have been used in Paget's disease and osteoporosis over the years. At about the same time as all this, he was offered the position of Chief of Endocrinology at Harvard University (Massachusetts General Hospital). After some thought he decided to accept this post, one of the most prestigious in American medicine and, as a result, the whole group would be moved, lock, stock and barrel, to Boston.

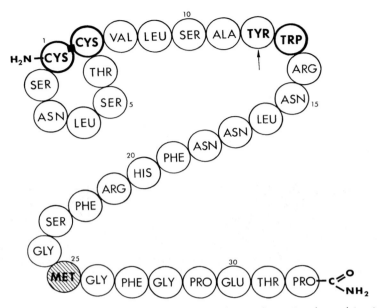

The chemical structure of the 32 aminoacid polypeptide porcine thyrocalcitonin.
Each ring represents an individual aminoacid, e.g. 1 is cystine; 32 proline amide
and so on.

I was offered a research post in Boston at the munificent salary of $30,000 a year, which might lead to an Assistant Professorship later. He was absolutely dumbfounded when, having thanked him politely, I declined. I cobbled together some excuse about dependent relatives in the United Kingdom which I am sure that he found less than convincing. The real reasons were more complex. Judith and I had no wish to settle in America. We found the whole society mercenary and materialistic. Moreover, racist attitudes towards the blacks were still commonplace in Maryland. Finally, Martin Luther King had been assassinated in April 1968 and Robert Kennedy would share the same fate in the Summer. In short, this society had, in the past, killed the red man and enslaved the black man; and now was in the process of assassinating its leaders!

A minor episode illustrates the contrast very well. Len Deftos and I were on the landline to the computer in central Washington one day, shortly after Luther King was shot, when up came the message 'Owing to the civil disturbance in the City this service is temporarily suspended'. In

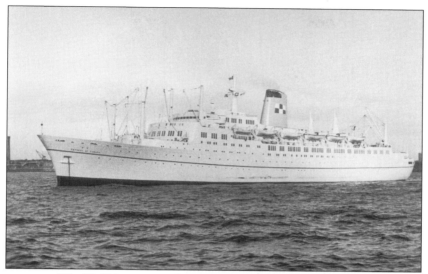

The RMS Empress of Canada *(photograph taken in 1961).*

fact, large-scale riots took place in the downtown area of Washington in the 'black' areas. As I drove home, the National Guard tanks were rolling down the main road into the blazing city.

We planned to return to the United Kingdom in early September but would leave, not from New York, but from Montreal on the *Empress of Canada*. I organized a route up through Pennsylvania (calling at Gettysburg), and onto the Great Lakes at Erie. We crossed into Canada at the Peace Bridge near Buffalo, where I called on the passengers in the car to sing, 'God Save the Queen' and 'The Maple Leaf for Ever'!

I had a nasty surprise at the Immigration Control on the Canadian side when I saw a notice that said, 'Canadian and American citizens straight on; other nationalities wait in line on left'. It turned out that our Canadian friends required an entry visa! After a lengthy interview and showing our tickets for berths on the ship, and the loading notice for the Austin 1100, the immigration officer very reluctantly gave us a holiday visa for two weeks and a dire warning as to the severe punishment that would ensure if we overstayed our welcome. The irony was that hundreds (if not thousands) of American draft dodgers were holed up in Canada at that time and some would try to get to Europe.

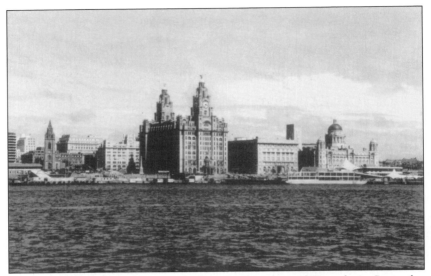

The Pier Head at Liverpool as seen from the Empress of Canada *in September 1968. The Liver building is in the centre of the picture. The natives return!*

After another tourist feast involving the Welland Canal, Niagara Falls, Fort Henry and the One Thousand Islands area of the St Lawrence River, we arrived in Montreal. Two days later we sailed for Glasgow and Liverpool. As Judith was putting the children to bed in the cabin, I sat in the bar, drinking a Manhattan and considering the year in America.

Scientifically it had been a worthwhile experience; I now knew how to develop a radio-immunoassay from scratch and this would prove valuable in the future. Politically and socially, I had purged myself of any desire to work in North America and when further offers came in from La Jolla, California, and other places, I was able to turn them down with confidence. After all they had no cricket and no football! I had missed Manchester United and in particular their winning the European Cup in 1968.

The future in Oxford was uncertain and I would be best advised to leave. I hoped to find a Senior Lectureship somewhere and build up my own research group. But where? Judith returned from looking after the children and we settled down to enjoy our cocoon-like existence for the next week in a great transatlantic liner.

CHAPTER 16

After Hubris Comes Nemesis: Disappointment in London (1968-1971)

Pride the never failing vice of fools.
Alexander Pope, 1688-1744
An essay on Criticism

WHEN WE ARRIVED back in the United Kingdom, things began to go wrong almost immediately. First there was a prolonged delay at the Customs in Liverpool to process the import of the Austin 1100. Then to cap matters with the car the gearbox began to overheat and had to be replaced, a sad indictment of British parts (and workmanship) after only 8,000 miles and twelve months ownership! When I reached Oxford (and the department) in mid September the atmosphere was quiet and gloomy. The Body Temperature group was closing and the technicians had left or were thinking about leaving. Bill Brown had wisely gone somewhat earlier to the new Hypertension Unit in Glasgow.

The first person I met on my return was the Unit Administrator, John Honour. He told me that in spite of all his years with the Regius, the first he had known about the translocation to Pembroke was when he read the announcement in the London *Times*! He was understandably disappointed by this and he awaited the appointment of a new Regius with anxiety as being in his mid-fifties he did not wish to move. I sympathized with him greatly and would have liked to stay but he understood clearly that I had to get out.

I sought an interview with the Regius in order to thank him for keeping my position open for a year. I had intended to tell him about the monograph that I was in the midst of writing on Renin and Hypertension but he then launched into a pep talk, 'Mike; if you're going to get a top job then you must do something that will receive general recognition'. I bit my tongue and forbore to tell him that I was better known outside Oxford than in it, for my work first on renin and now on thyrocalcitonin.

I left his office feeling that our relationship was at an end. I had to get out of the shadow of one of my giants, and try, as Joseph Conrad had expressed it so brilliantly, to cross the 'Shadow Line' to maturity.

There were two main possibilities: Nottingham (Tony Mitchell) or St Thomas's London (Bill Cranston). They had both recently been first assistants to Sir George. After some thought, I decided to approach Professor Cranston, who had a major interest in high blood pressure (as I did) and had intimated previously that there might be a post with him at St Thomas's. After some negotiation an offer of a Lectureship at St Thomas's came through and I moved to London in February 1969. This move proved problematic, as finding a house in London proved very difficult and the family could not transfer until the September. However, at last, we found a place to live in Thames Ditton, in an attractive area of Surrey close to Hampton Court and the Thames.

For the first nine months I had to stay with my cousin in Surbiton and go home to Oxford at the weekends. This was not only very unsatisfactory; it was exhausting. For some reason I was feeling very tired; I put it all down to post American gloom and the move to London but as I shall describe, it turned out to be more serious than that.

The only positive news in 1969 was the publication of my monograph 'Renin and Hypertension: A Modern Synthesis'. It was on the whole well received and I sent a copy to the Regius saying cheekily (and unwisely) that if I was to get a top job this is the sort of thing that I must do. Using the monograph I also used a loophole in the Oxford Doctor of Medicine regulations, to obtain this degree on published work.

My purpose at St Thomas's was to develop a radioimmunoassay for plasma renin activity but this was proving very difficult. I had no money for research and the laboratory was well equipped for animal experiments but not at all for work with radioactive isotopes. Peter Lewis joined me on a research fellowship and we set up an experimental model of hypertension in the rabbit but progress was painfully slow.

In 1970 two Senior Lectureships arose in the Department and I applied for one of these posts. To my severe disappointment I was not offered either of them. I realized my research progress had been very poor but setting up in a new laboratory where the techniques have not previously been used can take up to two years. I went through a period of great depression and disillusionment. I had largely done all that the system had

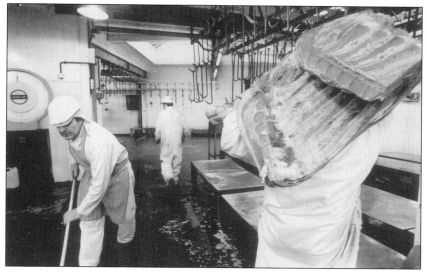

Smithfield Meat Market, London.
Weddel Pharmaceuticals was based about 400 yards away.

asked me to do; I had a national and international reputation, but I could not obtain a senior post in my own country whereas I had been offered jobs right, left, and centre in North America. Truly I felt that a prophet hath honour save in his own country! In these depths of gloom an offer came through the post from the Managing Director of Weddel Pharmaceuticals to become Medical Director of that company. I went over to Smithfield in the City to see him.

My interest had been aroused by the fact that Weddel was involved in the manufacture of natural products such as insulin and heparin and had recently made a 'breakthrough' in the treatment of gallstones. In the late 1960s, for an academic to join the pharmaceutical industry was regarded as the kiss of death. Drug firm doctors were regarded as no more (and no less) than the paid hirelings of the marketing department. In spite of all this, I took the impetuous decision to join Weddel and metaphorically to wipe the dust of St Thomas's from my feet! I told a colleague that I was selling my birthright for a mess of pottage; in fact for £6,000 a year, and a Triumph two-litre six-cylinder car! I went home to Thames Ditton on a beautiful autumn October day and I cleared up the garden for a very satisfactory bonfire, which included metaphorically all my vanities. Weddel would be my fourth professional address in two years. What had I done?

CHAPTER 17

Smithfield Market
(1971-1973)

But the jingling of the guinea
helps the hurt that Honour feels.
Alfred, Lord Tennyson 1809-1892

My welcome to Weddel Pharmaceuticals was in sharp contrast to that I had received at St Thomas's. I was the first physician to join the Management Team and my opinions were greeted with respect and often acted upon with alacrity, a refreshing contrast to life in Academic Medicine. Even more striking, I was immediately given a personal secretary which to a struggling Lecturer was riches beyond the dreams of avarice!

I answered to David Moreau who was the Managing Director. David was a compelling character: a Cambridge graduate who was fluent in several European languages, he had considerable personal charm. He loved the publicity side of the business and he informed me that our first task was to organize a conference on chenic acid (chenodeoxycholic acid) Weddel's new treatment to dissolve gallstones in situ in the gallbladder. This was indeed exciting as it was the first drug that could be given by mouth that had been shown to be able to exert such an effect. We hired a great hall and Professors Hofmann and Small who were leading pundits on the subject came over to speak from the United States. There was great excitement and it was widely reported in the Press.

It later turned out that only about 5% of gallstones would respond to the treatment. The stones must not be too big (or calcified) and they must be largely composed of cholesterol. From what we imagined would be a huge market, with major cash flows, the whole picture would shut down considerably. Weddel Pharmaceuticals faced other structural problems. It was a wholly owned subsidiary of Union International, a huge organization with many other offshoots including British Beef and Dewhursts the

111

**CHENODEOXYCHOLIC
ACID**

*The chemical structure of the primary bile acid chenodeoxycholic acid.
Chenos means goose and cholic bile (from the Latin).*

butchers. The company had never made a profit and it did not look like doing so. An expensive factory had been built in North Wales, at Wrexham, with state of the art machinery but full production had been delayed both by the necessary installation of a sprinkler system and disputes with the Transport and General Workers Union. Behind the scenes, David Moreau was in dispute with his superior, Oliver Philpott.

Weddel's other major problem was that it did not have its own dedicated research department and had to rely on that of the parent company. Chenic acid had been a lucky accident but promising leads were neglected which, in other peoples' hands, would lead to the low molecular weight heparins and the isolation of tumour necrosis factor and other inflammatory cytokines.

I now had other things to worry about apart from Weddel. One morning I was shaving; and on looking in the mirror noticed a lump in the neck, low down on the right side; lying on the muscle scalenus anterior. I felt it carefully; it was fairly mobile and non-tender and my

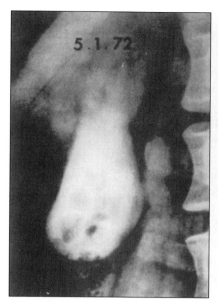 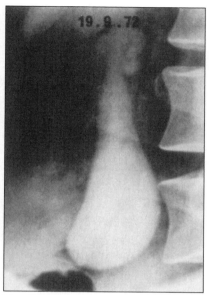

*A patient with gall stones in the gall bladder (left). They disappear in approxi-
mately eight months following oral treatment with the bile acid (right).*

clinical experience told me it was likely to be a lymph node. My diagnostic training suggested that the most likely possibilities were either
tuberculosis or a lymphoma (commonly Hodgkin's disease). I rang
Professor Semple at the Middlesex Hospital who was sceptical but asked
me to go to his outpatients (I was already working there doing an
occasional session).

His face changed when he felt the lump. 'It's an enlarged gland. You'll
have to come in to have it taken out'. He did not bother to tell me the
differential diagnosis as it was obvious: bad (tuberculosis) to much worse
(Hodgkin's disease). Microscopic examination would establish the truth. I
had it removed the next week and a few days later Professor Semple rang
me and said with some relief in his voice, 'Mike, it's tuberculosis! I am
putting you on a drug treatment regime which includes streptomycin,
isoniazid and para-amino-salicyclic acid (PAS)'. My thoughts flew back
four years (and three thousand miles) to Bethesda, Maryland, and the
Public Health Service physician. How stupid I had been not to take his
advice and use the prophylactic isoniazid!

Initially the treatment went well. The only side effect I noted, when Judith was giving me the streptomycin injection, was tingling round the mouth, a well-known side effect. However, other more serious problems were about to develop Every night, about 6 p.m. I began to have a rigor with violent shivering, accompanied by a temperature of 103°F, followed by profuse sweating. I would have to go to bed and by the next morning I would be fully recovered, only for the process to start all over again the next evening. After a week, the penny dropped; it was drug fever caused by PAS! I told Professor Semple; we stopped the PAS and the whole syndrome resolved. I took rifampicin (together with isoniazid) for the next twelve months and the infection was cured. Stephen and Karen received BCG (Bacille Calmette-Guérin) vaccine as a preventive injection.

Shortly after this, another bombshell exploded! I had been playing with the idea of looking for another position as I could see medium term problems for Weddel, unless it was sold to a bigger pharmaceutical company. Any idea of such a move was forestalled when, in December 1972, David Moreau called me into his office to say that he was leaving to become Managing Director of Elga Ltd (Water Softeners). This was surprising enough but more was to follow. Oliver Philpott was also to leave and he (David) had suggested to Mr Edmund Vestey, the Chairman of Union International, that I should become Managing Director of Weddel, and he had agreed! I was nonplussed, to put it mildly. I had moved from being a Lecturer in Medicine to being a Managing Director in the short space of twelve months. I intended to do what I could to stabilize Weddel but I did not see myself being there in the medium term. I achieved some success. The factory began to achieve its output targets. Cecil Foll, an experienced physician, was appointed to my vacancy and I moved chenic acid towards a product licence.

As I recovered from tuberculosis, I became increasingly aware that it was not satisfying to do research through surrogates and I still wanted to have a research team of my own. I had learnt a great deal in the pharmaceutical industry about interpersonal skills, organizing a secretary, and interview techniques. The time had not been wholly wasted but, as my full fitness returned, I must, if possible, move back into academic medicine.

In July 1973, I applied for a position in the secretariat of the

Committee on Safety of Medicines in London and, at the same time, also applied for the position of Senior Lecturer in Clinical Pharmacology at Leeds University Medical School. I was offered the first post (after interview) but delayed my acceptance until I had been to Leeds. I told my immediate colleagues at Weddel that I was going to Yorkshire to look into some promising research (a bare-faced lie) and stayed at the Queens Hotel, a five-star hotel in the City (as befitted a managing director)!

With my new found experience, derived from Weddel, I had prepared all the questions that I could think of including, 'How much will your salary reduce? Answer: 'From £6,500 to £3,000 per annum'. I waited for the crunch question and it came right at the end. 'Why did you leave a promising academic career and go to Weddel?' Answer: 'In the first place I had been offered the job and in the second I was not well. I had developed tuberculosis and I did not know whether I would be able to continue my academic career. My treatment with rifampicin and isoniazid continues'. I was appointed to the post as from November 1973. I had unexpectedly been given a second chance in academic medicine and this time I must not waste it by impatience or impetuosity.

I went back to London and told Edmund Vestey that I wanted to teach young people and pursue my own research. He accepted my departure reluctantly but with good grace. As luck would have it the property market went very flat for a number of months and the house in Surrey would not sell. This, coupled with the substantial fall in salary in moving back into Academia, was throwing us into debt. I had to borrow money from my father on an interest free basis but nevertheless I was happy as we drove into Leeds over the M62 motorway. I was once again doing what I wanted to do.

CHAPTER 18

Transfer to Leeds United:
Let the White Rose Flourish
(1973-1984)

Happy the man and happy he alone,
He who can call today his own,
He who, secure within, can say
Tomorrow do thy worst, for I have lived today.
John Dryden 1631-1700
Translation of Horace Bk III xxix

IN RETROSPECT, the period I was about to spend at Leeds was the most fulfilling of my whole career. This was in spite of a very bad spell during the first two years.

The main individuals with whom I interacted in my new position were Professor Derek Wood (the Dean of the Medical School), Professor Michael Barrett (Professor of Pharmacology) and Professor George McNicol (Professor of Medicine). A brief sketch of each is necessary as they were all to affect my work very considerably in the next ten years.

Derek Wood had been the Professor of Pharmacology but relinquished this post to become the Dean and his main task was to supervise the building of the new Medical School in the Worsley building. I took an immediate liking to him as he reminded me strongly of Uncle Willie (see Chapter 4). It then transpired, to my surprise and delight, that he had in fact been brought up in South Manchester, had attended William Hulme's School and then gone on to Brasenose College! For this reason he was biased in my favour and when, in time, good reports of my teaching came back, he became a strong supporter of mine. Very sadly, after he retired, he was struck down by motor neurone disease, terrible and rapidly fatal, which blighted his latter years.

Michael Barrett had come to the Department of Pharmacology from ICI Pharmaceuticals, at Alderley Park, Cheshire, where he had carried out very distinguished work on the ßeta-adrenergic blockers leading to the development of the lead compound atenolol. On reaching Leeds he had found a 'run down' department of Pharmacology, the state of which he blamed on neglect by the Dean, Derek Wood. There was not a single medically qualified person in the department and the medical students were constantly complaining that the teaching was not 'relevant' to the clinical course and their future work as doctors. My appointment was a step that had been taken to try and correct this deficiency which had also been noted by the University Grants Committee.

Professor George McNicol had arrived three years earlier to take the Chair of Medicine following the retirement of Ronald Tunbridge. A graduate and medallist of the University of Glasgow, he had led there an excellent group working on haemostasis and thrombosis. Transferring to Yorkshire must have been a culture shock and the Department of Medicine was also in a poor state. The only good thing to be said for it was that it was in a new block, the Martin wing and had an excellent suite of offices and laboratories.

My post was to be divided: fifty percent of my time to be spent in Pharmacology and fifty percent in Medicine. I had two laboratories, one in each department. I realized immediately that this was a recipe for disaster as in 'split' posts you must antagonize one master or the other.

Initially I decided to concentrate on the teaching while I assessed the research position. I had responsibilities in the second and third years in Pharmacology and the fifth year in Therapeutics. I organized a special course in the latter subject for the final year students in medicine, in which I hammered home to them, by the Socratic method, basic facts about the Materia Medica and the treatment of common conditions. The course was very successful and I had unsolicited thanks from a number of students and a few wrote letters to the Dean praising the course (which was almost unheard of in his experience). He conveyed his thanks to me personally and in his eyes I became virtually fireproof!

Michael Barrett initially welcomed me with open arms but as time went on and my clinical responsibilities increased, I found that I could not spend half of my time in Pharmacology. Over the years he complained to the Dean a number of times about this but Derek Wood took no notice at all of these complaints because of his personal dislike of Professor Barrett and also the way I had transformed the fifth year teaching.

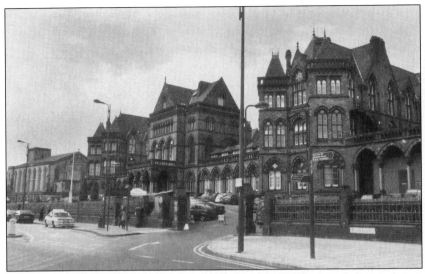

The Leeds General Infirmary, Great George Street. The frontal elevation.

This problem between Michael Barrett and myself led to a prolonged 'stand-off' and would in the course of time lead to my leaving Leeds some ten years later. One night after we had had a few beers together, he told me that he had been turned down for medical school entry by Guy's Hospital at the age of eighteen years and this had rankled with him ever since. This may have partially explained his attitude to doctors, in general, and to me, in particular!

I also had to build up an area of clinical expertise once again and I settled on renal disease and hypertension. Publications followed on sodium losing pyelonephritis; phaeochromocytoma; Gordon's syndrome (familial hypertension with hyperkalaemia) and fibromuscular hyperplasia of the renal arteries. We were fortunate to have in Leeds Professor Geoffrey Giles (a noted vascular surgeon) who operated very successfully on my patients. Sadly he died prematurely after I had left Leeds for Edinburgh. I also achieved one great diagnostic coup! Professor McNicol admitted a French boy with recurrent febrile attacks and I was asked to see him. The story only fitted one disorder, that of Familial Mediterranean Fever (FMF) and so it proved. I had never seen a case of FMF but I had worked in America with others who had.

My main problem was to find a long term research project in relation to the kidney and hypertension. Professor McNicol had generously provided me with the basic costs of setting up a laboratory. I had missed out on four years of advance in the renin/angiotensin field. In any case, the Glasgow group under Lever, Robertson and Brown (and others) had this area of research all sewn up. Radioimmunoassay for renin activity had become commercially available. It would be of no use to pursue that line.

A chance remark by Michael Barrett gave me the opening that I had been looking for and would start a twenty year research programme: 'Why is there so much dopamine in urine?' I do not believe he realized the full implication of what he was saying but, as Louis Pasteur once said, chance favours the prepared mind and a couple of days later the answer came to me like a flash of lightning! Dopamine must be formed in the kidney and as a powerful vasodilator could influence sodium handling and arterial blood pressure. This takes but a moment to say but it was to take five years to prove and twenty years to develop.

Fortunately I was joined by Stephen Ball, now Professor of Cardio-vascular Medicine at the University of Leeds, as my first Research Fellow and we were able to develop the idea. He was followed by a succession of able and enthusiastic individuals including Nicholas Oates, Michael Perkins, Ian Casson, John Harvey and David Worth. It became possible to show that dopamine is indeed synthesized in the kidney from L-dopa; that its formation is increased by sodium (but not potassium) loading; and that its production is blunted in chronic renal failure and essential hypertension. We were helped in these studies by having access to a fine metabolic ward where the diet of our volunteers (and patients) could be closely controlled.

As a result of this work, I became once again well known and was asked to speak in America, Canada, and all over Europe. I was also recognized by my fellow physicians when I was elected FRCP (London) in 1977 and at about the same time became a member of the Association of Physicians of Great Britain and Ireland. The Merit award system with its freemasonry began to work and I, mysteriously, became the proud possessor of a 'C' award and then a 'B'. For the first time since leaving America in 1968, I was free of money worries. It had taken a long time! By then I was 45 years old and did not have the benefits of private practice.

The chemical structure of the catecholamine dopamine
(3,4-dihydroxyphenylethylamine) and its N-methyl derivative epinine.

Another very positive feature of the Leeds General Infirmary was the Consultants' Dining Room. Here I would go for lunch and meet with kindred spirits such as Malcolm Parsons (Neurology), Julian Roberts (Psychiatry), Kenneth Exley (Neurophysiology) and 'Pip' Silk (Orthopaedics). It was very like a gentleman's club; there were very few female consultants. Tension was relieved and I learned a great deal from consultants in other subjects together with essential hospital gossip. I also developed very good relations with my two consultant colleagues in the Department of Medicine, John Wales (Diabetes) and Andrew Davies (Haemostasis and Thrombosis).

I intended to stay at Leeds until I retired as everything was going along extremely well but this gilded period could not last and it did not. From 1982 onwards, a number of events occurred, both personal and professional, which would lead inevitably and sadly to my leaving Leeds. The first was my father's death in 1982. Mother had died previously of metastatic colonic cancer (in 1975) and father had battled on heroically in Manchester, living alone. He began to fail and then in September 1982, I was summoned home from a conference in Oxford by a telephone message to say he was ill. I drove over to Manchester to find him confused and with markedly slurred speech. Within 24 hours he was admitted to my own hospital in Leeds. A CAT scan showed a large subdural haematoma and, in spite of a drainage operation by the neurosurgeons, he died 48 hours later.

Despite all the 'fights' I had had with him, between the ages of 18 and 25, we had now developed a great mutual respect and I realized that he was a product of his environment, times and customs. I found the arrangements for the cremation difficult to undertake and the whole week of the funeral I was very agitated. Some of this was the natural grief that one expects but as it would turn out later, it was to prove more than this. The day before the funeral I had to give an invited Lecture to a Regional Conference of the Royal College of Physicians at Leeds with Douglas Black (President) in the audience. How I got through it I will never know, but Douglas was good enough to mention me in his after dinner speech that same evening.

At about the same time, Frank Parsons, a distinguished renal physician and pioneer of renal dialysis who worked in the Infirmary suggested to Professor McNicol that I be put forward for a personal Chair as he was fearful that Leeds might lose me to Cardiff or Glasgow, where chairs of Clinical Pharmacology were about to become vacant. Professor McNicol agreed and supported the proposal strongly. It went forward to the University where, several months later, it was turned down. I had my suspicions as to the person (or persons), who had blocked it but I resolved not to let the decision rankle but to look for an opportunity to move elsewhere if a suitable position came up.

Early in 1983 I began to feel unwell. We used to walk the dog regularly in Roundhay Park on a Sunday morning and I started to feel short of breath on a particular ascent of Soldier's Field. I thought nothing much of it at the time nor did I take much notice of my hair going silvery white at around the same period. Judith had been troubled by my gradual change in temperament; I began to be irritable and bad tempered with the children (nouty as it is called in the North of England!). She was just about to ask for John Wales my colleague to help her with my problems, as she had noticed also that I was losing weight, when the situation declared itself, of all places, in the laboratory at work.

I was about to take part, as a normal volunteer, in yet another dopamine experiment, when John Harvey and David Worth (my research fellows) came in clutching some laboratory results including my own. John said rather sheepishly, 'Your blood count is abnormal. Your MCV (mean cell volume) is 108 cubic microns when the upper limit is 98!' The three of us knew there were two main diagnostic possibilities for this macrocytosis (large red cells); heavy intake of alcohol or deficiency of haematinic factors such as B_{12} or folate! The news reverberated like a thunderclap. I said, 'It's got to be pernicious anaemia! My mother had it!'

And so it proved! I went to see Brian Roberts, a Consultant Haematologist, who after further tests confirmed the diagnosis of pernicious anaemia. Judith asked why it was called pernicious and I told her that, before liver extract and B_{12}, it used to kill people in about five years, from cardiac failure, often combined with serious neurological damage (subacute combined degeneration of the spinal cord). I also took home some ampoules of vitamin B_{12} (a beautiful dark red – from the cobalt it contained), syringes and needles.

Judith had not given an injection for some time but in went the B_{12}, initially three times a week. I wondered whether I would get the classical B_{12} euphoria combined with a burst of energy. To my delight, after about a week, I had a real blast of enthusiasm and started to reconstruct the garden. The breathlessness disappeared rapidly, excessive sleepiness went and within three months my grey hair had gone dark again. One symptom (or problem) was more recalcitrant and lasted several years. I started to get panic attacks, and with these, anticipatory anxiety of flying, busy roads, crowded stores and some committees. I learned that B_{12} deficiency can present with neuropsychiatric syndromes such as dementia, depression, anxiety and panic attacks.

At about the same time as my illness developed, Professor McNicol took us into his office and announced that he was going to Aberdeen University, as Principal and Vice-Chancellor. This was a blow but not wholly unexpected. It would presage another period of uncertainty, as had happened to me before, when Sir George Pickering retired. I had come over the years to admire and respect Professor McNicol greatly. Initially I was slow to warm to him as he seemed reserved and somewhat authoritarian but as I grew to know him better I realized that he was a superb administrator with a pawky sense of humour.

He kindly agreed to act as my referee after he had moved to Aberdeen and this was to prove crucial later. My first decision was whether or not to apply for the Chair of Medicine which he had vacated. With some reluctance I decided to do so, knowing full well that Leeds had always been reluctant to appoint internal candidates. A classic example was my friend Michael Green, a fine forensic pathologist, who had to go to Sheffield to find a Chair! My prognostications proved correct. I did not even get an interview although a friend on the Appointments Committee told me later that many had wanted to see me. Colin Prentice from

Glasgow was appointed to the position. He was and is an expert on haemostasis and thrombosis and would continue the work (and the group) started by Professor McNicol. My friends in the Consultants' dining room were disappointed as was Professor Verna Wright (rheumatologist; now sadly dead) as he had written a personal letter of recommendation to the Dean. I had now been turned down both for a personal Chair and that in Medicine. It was time to go!

Three chairs came up in quick succession; Dundee, Leicester and Edinburgh. Dundee was the first to interview; the short list was Lee, McDevitt (Belfast) and Prescott (Edinburgh). I was very much the outsider and Dr McDevitt was appointed. Ironically I would join Laurie Prescott (at Edinburgh) within about a year! The second short list was at Leicester and here the inside candidate David Barnett was appointed. I had a good interview and the external assessor was Professor James Robson of Edinburgh (Medicine) and he questioned me closely and extensively.

In early February 1984 came the interviews for Edinburgh. I was relaxed about the process because Colin Prentice had told me that if this application went down, he would put me forward again for a Personal Chair at Leeds. In fact I was so laid-back that I went into James Thin's bookshop, opposite the Old College on South Bridge, and bought the life of the great scientist Ernest Rutherford while I was waiting for the interview. It stands on my shelves to this day as a memorial to that fateful February occasion.

I was summoned into the room by Professor Burnett, the Vice-Chancellor, who made to me a more or less offhand remark, 'Ah, you're the one who worked in industry'. I replied without thinking, 'Yes – I am the spy who came in from the cold'. This caused a few laughs around the table; broke the ice and I was away and running. The first external assessor was Professor William Paton, who was Head of Pharmacology at Oxford (and Bill Cook's boss). Here, chance (and fortune) came to my aid. He said as an opening gambit, 'Your first reference in your curriculum vitae is to Dr W F Cook and yourself.' I said, 'Yes, it was in the RPM Dept. at Oxford'. Immediately he knew that we had met and he also knew of my contribution to the renin/angiotensin system. After that, growing in confidence, I dispatched questions in all directions, apart from one nasty one from the Dean of Medicine, Professor Gordon Whitby who said, 'Is your health good?' I replied, 'Yes, it is'. This was the truth but not the whole truth – I should have replied, 'Yes, on B12'!

The hour long interrogation had passed, as it were, in the blink of an eye. I walked quickly down over the North Bridge to Waverley Station and took the East Coast Main Line to York and then on to Leeds. I did not know whether I would get the job but at least I had acquitted myself reasonably well. The next morning a letter arrived offering me the Chair. I replied by return, accepting the position but on the understanding I could transfer my 'B' merit award to Edinburgh. I was not going to take a substantial cut in salary again. I had done so twice before, once on returning from America, and a second time on leaving Weddel Pharmaceuticals for Leeds!

The Dean also wrote to me asking if I had any specific requirements. I knew it would be counter-productive to ask for more Lecturers (or a bigger departmental budget) as Edinburgh, like most other British Universities at that time was facing severe financial retrenchment. I asked simply if I could transfer my Medical Laboratory Scientific Officer, Janet Brown, to Edinburgh. This was agreed. I asked also whether the Chair could be designated the Christison in honour of Robert Christison, a great Edinburgh physician and toxicologist. The Committee deemed this inappropriate! What did inappropriate mean?

At all events I had fallen, almost by default, into one of the most prestigious chairs of Clinical Pharmacology and Therapeutics in the country which had been held previously by such luminaries as Sir Robert Christison (the father of British Toxicology), Sir Thomas Fraser (who had isolated physostigmine and developed the idea of agonist and antagonist drugs) and Sir Derrick Dunlop (who had been largely responsible for the creation of the Committee on Safety of Medicines). I did not know whether I could do the job but I would give it my best shot. My only hope, after the scares with pernicious anaemia and tuberculosis, was that my state of health would not interfere prematurely with my efforts and I would manage a reasonable period in the post. I had never worked in Edinburgh, or indeed anywhere in Scotland. The University was appointing an outsider; would I be treated with friendliness or suspicion? Time alone would tell!

CHAPTER 19

North to Edinburgh: A Scottish Enlightenment (1984-1995)

Perhaps it is hardly desirable that an active man of science should obtain a chair too early, for I have noticed that the wood of which academic fauteuils are made, has a narcotic quality which occasionally renders the occupants somnolent, lethargic or even comatose!

Oliver Wendell Holmes to
Weir Mitchell (the Neurologist)
1864

I WAS APPOINTED to the Chair at Edinburgh in February 1984 but was not to go there until the October of the same year. This left me with an awkward period of eight months in which I existed in a kind of limbo; part neither of one place nor the other. My position was advertised and Morgan Feely, who had worked with me as a Lecturer, was promoted and brought his considerable experience in the treatment of epilepsy and work on compliance with drug therapy to the post. Within weeks there was also to be an ironic development. It was announced that Michael Barrett had been appointed Vice-Chancellor of the private University of Buckingham. The long stand-off we had experienced would be resolved, not by one of us leaving, but indeed by both!

Derek Wood made a generous gesture to myself (and Judith) when he, and his wife, invited us for a day to his Pennine cottage. The weather was perfect, as only a June day in England can be, and the whole experience had an elegiac quality. I knew that I would probably never see him again and it felt somewhat like parting from a relative. As I drove away from the cottage to go back to Leeds, I reflected on the vagaries of chance that had thrown two Manchester and Brasenose men together.

In the intervening months of the interregnum, I made several visits to the Department in Edinburgh. I also met with Laurie Prescott (Reader and Acting Head), Professor James Robson (Medicine) and Professor Gordon Whitby (Dean of Medicine).

Laurie Prescott, who had been a candidate for the Chair, was understandably disappointed after being passed over. I sympathized with him totally as this had happened to me at Leeds, not once but twice. I hoped he would stay in Edinburgh, as we needed his expertise on paracetamol toxicity and poisoning in general. In these areas he was a recognized international authority. I was therefore pleased when Gordon Whitby suggested that he put Laurie forward for a personal Chair and I gave this proposal my wholehearted support. Within about twelve months this well merited promotion came through.

The Dean, Gordon Whitby, was a difficult man to get to grips with. I had already had one brush with him over the 'Christison' title for the Chair and I would not find him easy to negotiate with. He tended to address individuals as if talking to a public meeting. Nevertheless, as Professor of Clinical Chemistry, he was not constrained by duties to patients and therefore had more time to devote to administrative chores. His much busier clinical colleagues were therefore 'happy' to see him carry out two consecutive terms of office as it got them off the hook. Eventually he and I reached a modus vivendi! Indeed he became a strong supporter of mine. Professor Robson was in his early sixties and had had a distinguished career as a nephrologist. Once he had seen me in post for twelve months he decided to retire and Professor Ian Bouchier (from Dundee University) took his place after a gap of twelve months.

The Department of Clinical Pharmacology was dispirited when I arrived. Professor Ronald Girdwood, the previous incumbent, had retired in October 1982 and at first no money could be found to replace him. After some time Squibb Pharmaceuticals, of Princeton, New Jersey, not only guaranteed my salary but also gave me a substantial research grant for seven years. The first task I had was to try and lift corporate spirits after the prolonged and damaging interregnum. I summoned the two lecturers, Dr Julian Critchley and Dr Stephen Freestone, and told them that if they wanted to leave then I would help them in any way I could but I hoped they would stay. I also told them that we had money from the Wellcome Trust to appoint a further Lecturer and, shortly afterwards, Dr Tom MacDonald joined us from Dundee University. Fortunately two central

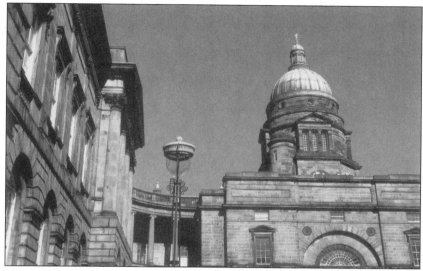

The main quadrangle and tower of the Old College at the University of Edinburgh.

figures had carried over from Professor Girdwood's tenure: Dick Samson the Senior Chief Technician and Elspeth Shields, the Administrative Secretary. Both were to prove towers of strength in the coming days, months and years. Janet Brown, my MLSO from Leeds, joined us after about six months, and was to prove extremely valuable in setting up my research effort.

The first major test of my incumbency was the Inaugural Lecture! Largely abandoned by other universities, Edinburgh has persisted with this trial by ordeal. I had lectured all over the world but to address one's future colleagues (and the general public) made even the strongest quail.

I had heard one or two inaugural lectures and mostly they were boring as people read from prepared notes. I decided to go for broke and have only a short prepared introduction (and close) but rely for the major part on extempore delivery prompted by transparent slides as aides memoire. This was a high-risk strategy!

The great day came. The Principal Dr Burnett introduced me to the serried ranks in the Old Anatomy Theatre and I set off. By great good fortune the Muse of Oratory took over; no doubt propelled by high octane adrenaline. The fifty minutes passed as if on wings and I do not remember the thanks of the Principal (or the applause). We then processed out into the anteroom for the reception. I did not know (and often this is the case) whether the Lecture had been good, bad or indifferent. However as Professor Bernard Ginsborg (Pharmacology) said as he was leaving, 'That was a splendid inaugural!' I realized that I had made a definite impact. I was exhausted but the high risk strategy had paid off! Only on a few occasions has the Muse come to my aid and when it does it is almost like a dream or, as the psychiatrists would say, a fugue like state.

Once this ordeal was over I was able to assess my responsibilities in clinical work; teaching and research. At first my administrative responsibilities were limited. The wards assigned to us were 23 and 24 on the general medical corridor and the consultant team comprised myself, Prescott, Heading (Gastroenterology), Watson (General Medicine and Nephrology) and Ludlam (Haematology). I have always welcomed meeting new colleges and I learnt about the oesophagus from Bob Heading; polycystic disease of the kidneys from Michael Watson; and haemophilia (and other bleeding disorders) from Chris Ludlam. I also joined the Hypertension Clinic with Michael Watson and Sandy Muir. My teaching burden was less than at Leeds and I had very little preclinical responsibilities in Pharmacology which was a relief.

The main problem I had was the effort that would be required, for the fifth time in my career (Oxford, Washington, London, Leeds and now Edinburgh) to set up a research programme. I decided that the Leeds radioisotope method for dopamine measurement was too cumbersome. Employing Dick Samson's expertise we set up a high pressure liquid chromatography (HPLC) method which could process many more samples in unit time. Janet Brown set up the plasma renin activity method and also raised antibodies to atrial natriuretic factor which led to a radioimmunoassay for this substance. Unfortunately, there was no Metabolic Unit in the Royal Infirmary. As a result this type of study, which had been so successful at Leeds, would not be possible. We therefore concentrated on studying prodrugs for dopamine (that is a drug which would release dopamine in the kidney). After some time we concentrated our efforts on Y-L-glutamyl-L-dopa, which was to give us ten years of work on the kidney. It was a disappointment that this drug could not be given by mouth as it is rapidly destroyed by the stomach, intestine and liver. To this day, unfortunately, there is only one good peripheral dopamine agonist (fenoldopam) and this also has to be given intravenously.

The research output of our Department picked up rapidly and our papers published, to research worker ratio, exceeded that of the Department of Medicine for several years. Further support was gained from the National Kidney Research Foundation and private individuals. The Winthrop Foundation also funded a visiting Lecturer and several international figures came to see us, subsidized by this financial support. As one Lecturer (or Research Fellow) left, others came to replace them. Julian Critchley went to a Chair in Hong Kong but was tragically killed in a road accident in 2001. Tom MacDonald is now a Professor of Clinical Pharmacology in Dundee. Robin Jeffrey, Stephen Hutchison, and Emile Li Kam Wa came in to replace them. All three have now gone on to consultant posts in Bradford, Inverness and Blackpool respectively.

Gradually my administrative responsibilities began to expand, not because I wished it but people became aware of my skills in this area (derived to a degree from my managerial experience at Weddel). This culminated in my becoming Chairman of the Department of Medicine (on a rotating basis). My period of office coincided with the first running of the Research Assessment exercise (RAE) by the University Grants Committee. This would decide the funding of the British Universities over the next four years. It was a mammoth task and I spent six months focusing almost entirely on this important return. On our efforts depended literally millions of pounds of grants in aid. There was widespread rejoicing when we were placed in the highest category and I received a letter of thanks from the Dean, who by then, was Professor Christopher Edwards.

The tasks multiplied: examining in MB.Ch.B; MRCP (UK); Ph.Ds all over the country; refereeing papers for Clinical Science and the British Journal of Clinical Pharmacology; designing a new course in Clinical Skills and an examination to assess it. The burdens seemed endless and the clinical load increased inexorably as the number of acute beds in other hospitals in Edinburgh fell progressively. Towards the end of my tenure it was not at all unusual to take in 40 to 50 acute medical admissions in 24 hours; far too many to maintain an excellent standard of care for all. Probably our greatest success in retrospect was to persuade Syntex to fund a Clinical Research Unit at the Western General Hospital and then to recruit David Webb to be the director. As will be seen, he was to take over the Chair from me in 1995.

There was to be one final Eureka moment! Between 1992 and 1995, Dr Emile Li Kam Wa using Y-L-glutamyl-5-hydroxytryptophan was able to establish that there were 5-hydroxytryptamine (5-HT) receptors in the kidney and these may well be important in disease states such as glomerulonephritis and other disorders of that organ. I had intended to go on until 65, the usual retiring age, but the Blind Fury was once more to intervene and force a change of plan as it had threatened to do before, both in London and Leeds.

CHAPTER 20

Illness and Retirement
(1995-2003)

I am expected to be scientist and committee man; artist; official;
benefactor; doctor and invalid! I am up to my neck in stacks of
screed for various committees, scrawling over all kinds of reports,
notifications, memoranda, recommendations and decisions. A heap
of utter rubbish! Lord, when will it all end?

Borodin – Professor of Organic Chemistry
and Distinguished Composer (1827)
St Petersburg

As I approached sixty years of age, I began to feel tired; not the
indescribable tiredness of pernicious anaemia but a general
frustration with the reams of paper passing across my desk, in particular
the questionnaires coming from the University, the National Health
Service and other august bodies. My views began to resemble those
quoted from Borodin!

With my medical history, I knew that I was sailing into the minefields
and I wondered idly, from time to time, when I would strike a problem.
As it turned out within twelve months of my fifty-eighth birthday,
three difficulties came together: bladder neck obstruction; cataract and
glaucoma; and a transient cerebral ischaemic attack.

Recurrent urinary tract infection had led to a fibreoptic endoscopic
examination which showed not the expected prostatic hypertrophy but
narrowing of the urethra at the entrance to the bladder. This was dilated
under local anaesthesia and I have never experienced such pain in my life!
I sympathized with the old surgeon who prayed every night that, 'when
thou takest me Lord, take me not through the bladder'.

Shortly after this I noticed glare, when driving at night, and was
referred to Mr Bartholomew at the Eye Pavilion where I was found to
have a post-traumatic cataract (and glaucoma) in the right eye; the one
that had been damaged by gang warfare in childhood. This led to an

intraocular lens implant and a drainage operation. The field of vision improved but the pressure rose again, after five years. The right eye now requires timolol and prostaglandin eye drops to keep the pressure under control.

The most frightening episode occurred while I was chairing a meeting of the Physicians' Committee. I suddenly felt very dizzy; my left side felt heavy and my left arm became incoordinate. I had to leave the meeting and go home. The diagnosis was either a brain stem transient ischaemic attack or a small lacunar infarct in the same area. Happily the problem cleared up in two or three days but it was found that my blood pressure was running between 180/100 and 190/110 mms Hg. As a result, I am now on lifelong treatment with diuretic and ß-adrenergic blocker. Aspirin was also started in an attempt to stop further ischaemic events in the brain. After a while, this caused occult gastrointestinal bleeding and I have now been switched to clopidogrel, another antithrombotic agent, which so far I seem to tolerate very well.

These three events persuaded me to think about retirement, as two of them (the eye and the blood pressure) would certainly be long-term problems. I do not think (or at least I hope) that my consultant colleagues had noticed any marked deterioration in my performance in respect of clinical duties but the writing was on the wall. I thought, to use the well-known phrase, rather go five minutes early than five years too late! I had seen too many professors (and heads of department) immobile in their chairs, obviously deteriorating and yet clinging on to office.

One Sunday afternoon, as I was driving into the Royal Infirmary to do the four o'clock ward round, I thought suddenly, 'It is enough'. I went home and discussed it with Judith. We had already gone over the possibility in general terms and she was worried about what I would do in the future but realized that I was now intent. On the Monday following, I sought an audience with the Dean, Professor Christopher Edwards, to convey my decision. I gave eighteen months notice, in order, I hoped, that the damaging hiatus that had occurred after Professor Girdwood's retirement could, in this instance, be avoided.

I had never forgotten how George Pickering's retirement had not been divulged to his dedicated staff but had come to them through the newspapers. I therefore went straight back to the Department and informed Laurie Prescott, Elspeth Shields and Dick Samson. I also told

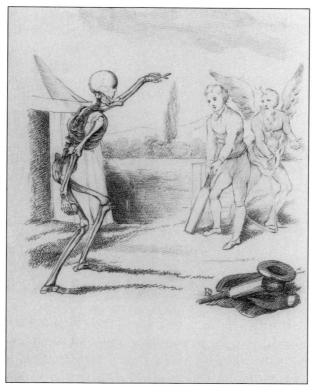

Death bowls and Father Time (with scythe) keeps wicket. From Death and the Cricketer in Death's Doings by Dagley. (See text and bibliography.)

my two lecturers, Stephen Freestone and Emile Li Kam Wa, as again, I wanted them to hear the news straight from me and not through the medium of the University Bulletin or that false jade rumour!

There were of course scientific papers to be finished and Dr Li Kam Wa's PhD thesis to be completed and examined. All of this went through successfully. The Department of Clinical Pharmacology would in time move to the Western General Hospital, a better place for it, and David Webb became the Professor without any delay. I was very annoyed when the Faculty called the position the Christison Chair which Gordon Whitby (and his committee) had refused to do for me eleven years earlier! However, life is unequal and unfair!

I left the department quietly in late September 1995. Would there be life after the Infirmary and Clinical Medicine? I had little time to think about this as immediately Michael Mitchell of Astra Pharmaceuticals in Edinburgh offered me part-time work and this was continued by Anne Lennon his successor. For two to three years, I enjoyed this enormously as I had power without responsibility (the prerogative of the harlot through the ages!). After this period, my right eye began to be troublesome as the intraocular pressure rose yet again and I retired for the second time in 1998. I now content myself with writing on medical history and the poisonous and medicinal plants. I have much more time to continue my book collecting activities, which include the illustrated children's books of Rackham and Dulac, and volumes and prints on the sport of cricket.

I have no regrets. To quote Horace, '*Pallida Mors aequo pulsat pede pauperium tabernas regiumque turres*' or in translation, 'Pale Death kicks with impartial foot at the door of poor men's cabins and regal towers' or in view of my lifelong interest in cricket, 'Death is bowling and Father Time is keeping wicket'. My wicket is still, for the moment, intact, but it is inevitable sooner or later that I will be given Out, Caught Time, Bowled Death! I have already survived several appeals for Leg Before Wicket!

Since I retired, both the University and the National Health Service have become battlefields. The NHS staggers from one crisis to another and few young medical graduates would wish a career in Academia. At times, an honourable profession has also been brought low by scandal. We must hope that eventually both institutions will come through this vexatious period. It will not be an easy process.

CHAPTER 21

Reflections: What Does It All Mean?

Was du ererbt von deinen Vätern, erwirb es, um es zu besitzen.
What you have inherited from your forefathers, acquire it in order
to possess it.

J.W. Goethe

IN THIS SHORT MEMOIR, I have sought to emphasize the impact and
long-lasting influence that four very different individuals have had on
my professional life and the development of my career as a doctor and
scientist. The first of my role models (or giants) was Eric James. At first to
an undeveloped twelve year old he was a frightening Olympian figure but
when later, as a sixth former, I came to know him somewhat better, two
things about him impressed me very greatly. The first was his great
determination to strive for excellence in many areas of school life and
activity; and the second was his personal crusade to emphasize the
importance of education both for the individual and to society in general.
I have tried to carry forward both these principles in my career as a
physician and a university teacher. It is also of interest that in 1953, James
recommended that I should seek to go to St Mary's Hospital, London, for
my clinical training where he knew George Pickering was at that time!
Here lies an invisible thread that links people of distinction.

My second mentor was Douglas Black who influenced me in several
different ways. He, together with Bill Stanbury, were the first examples I
had encountered of that rare breed, the clinical academic, who combined
clinical medicine, teaching and research. Fired by their examples, I
determined that I would pursue such a post as a career objective and also,
if it were possible and an opportunity arose, I would seek to prosecute
clinical research on the kidney.

My third great role model was Archie Cochrane. From the outset, I
found him fascinating. His views on medicine chimed in with mine when
he expressed his antiestablishment and antiauthoritarian attitudes. He also

strongly encouraged me to go on asking questions even when my superiors regarded such questioning as inappropriate or, at times, impertinent. Archie has been criticized by some of his colleagues in that, as a bachelor of independent means, he could afford to hold controversial views and could let his career evolve come what may. There is truth in this but of all the four men, he had the greatest overall effect on modern medical practice. On a personal level he was a charming, amusing individual and as the Scots would say, a kenspeckled figure. Long after I had left Cardiff he was interested in the progression of my career.

The man who had the most impact on me and my career was George Pickering. He was a truly great clinical scientist and from him (and his staff) I was to learn how to pursue medical research and organize an investigative programme. By the time I came to know him in the 1960s, he was in constant pain from bilateral osteoarthritis of the hips and understandably he could be somewhat tetchy. As I have described, at a certain point I felt I had to break away from his influence and establish whether I could prosper as an independent research worker. This proved to be much more difficult that I had anticipated and led to a serious disappointment in London.

When I left Oxford I resolved that I would seek to supervise my own research group (however small). If I did, I would try and be as open and transparent with my staff as I could. I also realized that a therapeutic revolution was up and running and this would be based on basic scientific evidence. I resolved to be a part of this new wave. The years I spent in Sir George's Lane between 1961 and 1969 were the most formative of my career and I thank him for them.

As will have become clear in the course of this memoir, I came into medicine to find out about rheumatic fever and pernicious anaemia, the disorders which had affected me and my mother in the 1940s. Rheumatic fever has now largely disappeared in the United Kingdom although there have been recent outbreaks in the United States. Pernicious anaemia is still with us and it used to give me great pleasure to tell newly diagnosed patients in my own practice that I too had the disease; that it was eminently curable and that they would experience a period of B_{12} induced euphoria when treatment began.

It was a privilege and a pleasure to work as a clinical scientist for almost thirty years and to add a few drops of information to the vast sea of medical knowledge and therapy. As I sit now in my study in South Edinburgh, reflecting on the chances that threw me into the paths of these four distinguished individuals, I am reminded of the artist Lowry who repeatedly said to his friend Professor Hugh Maitland, 'What is it all for? What does it all mean?'

The first thing that has to be said is that luck, chance, or fate, plays a major part in all our lives although we are very reluctant to admit it. Two bouts of rheumatic fever damaged my heart but on the other hand determined my choice of medicine as a career. Later on, as I approached 50 years, I developed pernicious anaemia as a genetic legacy from my mother. I had no control over either of these events. Luck then plays a further part; the rheumatic mitral valvular disease of the heart has not yet killed me (sixty years on) although it could eventually do so; pernicious anaemia, at one time fatal, is now easily controlled by regular intra-muscular cobalamin (B_{12}). Pernicious anaemia came down from my mother's, the Radcliffe, line and essential hypertension down that of the Lees, the latter to declare itself about ten years ago. There is a compelling irony in that this disorder, that I had worked on for a number of years, has now come to claim me!

Apart from the genetic tendencies towards diseases (or disorders) I have also inherited certain characteristics which have been sometimes beneficial, sometimes deleterious. On the positive side a very good memory, enthusiasm and resilience; on the negative side, laziness, arrogance and impetuosity. At times, I have acted too hastily when mature reflection would have been more helpful, as in the saga of the positive Mantoux test and the glandular tuberculosis. A natural distrust of authority and those exercising it was manifest from my early days. This attitude of, 'I'll show them' resulted in conflict with my mentors on a number of occasions. I have also spoken out with too much candour and erred on the side of calling a spade a spade, and sometimes a bloody shovel! This forthrightness, a Mancunian trait, often irritated my superiors and I would have been better advised to proceed with more caution.

Of course my career has had its full measures of both successes and failures. For a time the medical academic system (and my own deficiencies) hindered my progress and diverted me into the pharma-ceutical industry. This interlude was not, as it turned out, a complete waste of time and I learned how to handle groups of people and exercise authority. I shall always be grateful for the second chance I was given at Leeds University by Derek Wood and others.

What abiding lessons have my education and career bequeathed? The first and most compelling imperative is to spend more money on education in all its phases. As I have pointed out earlier this was realized by Cobden and the Manchester School in the 1830s but he was then a voice crying in the wilderness. Belatedly nearly two hundred years later we are attempting to address the problem. In parallel with this we must recognize and honour teachers of all categories and express this appreciation with tangible rewards.

The second point that I would make is that the National Health Service, once the envy of the civilized world, was allowed to deteriorate sharply for a period of at least ten years. It now needs a continuum of guaranteed investment to bring us up to the standards of our Continental neighbours. The additional beds, doctors, nurses and ancillary workers cannot be simply conjured out of the air. If this means increasing the Standard Rate of Income Tax then so be it! After all, the Chancellor of the Exchequer now claims that we are the fourth largest economy in the world.

Turning now to my own personal credo, I have with reluctance abandoned traditional Christian belief in the sense that I can no longer accept (or believe) the Incarnation and the Resurrection. As a consequence, I can no longer affirm the Nicene or Athanasian creeds. If Jesus is simply a great prophet amongst other prophets what then are we left with? And yet, and yet! There is no doubt that Christian values (and their ethical consequences) have motivated many individuals to carry out countless works of self-sacrifice which even at times determined their own deaths. In answer to this paradox I have developed my own philosophy which involves Stoicism for oneself and Samaritanism to others.

To take Stoicism first, which I would also join with William Osler's equanimity: we will all face inevitably, in our private and professional lives, a time of trial. In my own case, I have had to face a number of illnesses and a serious eye injury. Judith and I also sustained the sad loss of an infant daughter with spina bifida and hydrocephalus. To maintain my continued good 'health', I now receive intramuscular vitamin B_{12}; and by mouth beta-adrenergic blockers, thiazide diuretic, clopidogrel, thyroxine; and two different eye drops for glaucoma.

Rather than ask, 'Why me?' the Stoic should ask, 'Why not me?' In fact I give thanks for all those physicians and scientists who, over the last two hundred years since the Scientific Enlightenment, worked so hard to make all these modern treatments possible. Of course, I recognize that the Blind Fury will account for me one day. Meanwhile, I ask like E. W. Fowler, the noted English lexicographer (who also had serious problems with his eyes) that I shall die before I go blind. Until this last I seize each day and continue with my literary efforts. Two quotations come often to mind which provide some consolation. The first is from Shakespeare's *Macbeth*, 'Come what, come may. Time and the hour runs through the roughest day' and the second is the motto from the Arms of Man. '*Quocunque jeceris stabit* – Whithersoever you may have thrown it, it will stand'.

The second pillar of my makeshift philosophy is that of Samaritanism. When Jesus was asked, 'Who is my neighbour?' after his injunction to love thy neighbour as thyself, he replied to the question from the lawyer by telling the parable of the Good Samaritan. When the man, going down from Jerusalem to Jericho, fell among thieves, help came not from the Jew, who passed by on the other side but from a Samaritan (regarded by them as a member of an unclean caste). Jesus then asked the further question, 'Who then was neighbour to this man who fell among thieves?' The reluctant answer came back from the disciples that it was the 'outcast', the Samaritan. It is often forgotten that Jesus ends the parable with the famous command, 'Go and do thou likewise!' or as the Latin has it in the Vulgate, '*Vade et fac similiter!*' It is no surprise that this is the motto of many nursing schools and colleges.

The idea of Samaritanism has been picked up and developed by the American author, Walsh McDermott in his thought-provoking essay Technology's Consort published in 1983. He emphasizes that doctors should use every technical and therapeutic advance that we can mobilize in our care for patients, but we must also bring to bear our emotional support for the individual. This additional support for the patient he calls Samaritanism. Of course this love and care has been deployed by the best nurses from time immemorial.

This variant of the Golden Rule, to treat thy neighbour as thyself, has

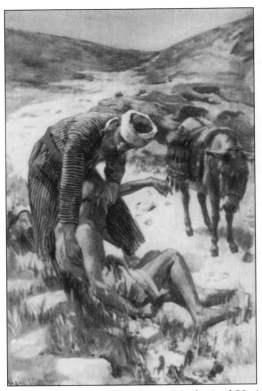

The Parable of the Good Samaritan King James (Authorized Version) of the Bible. Gospel according to Luke; Chapter X; verses 30 to 34. After a watercolour by Harold Copping.

echoed down the centuries from many philosophers and divines. In a recent treatment of the subject, McCormick in his book entitled 'The Doctor: Father Figure or Plumber?' has emphasized that the price for our peculiar privileges as physicians is the unremitting service we must give to our patients.

In the last fifty years the scientific juggernaut has threatened to take over the ancient art of the physician. Talking to patients and their relatives is tending to become a forgotten skill amongst the everyday pressures of targets, audit, research and teaching assessments. It is imperative that we inculcate the right attitudes into medical students, and young doctors in training, in order that they can communicate with patients (and their relatives) properly. To paraphrase the late Lord Platt of Rusholme it is just as important, if not more important, what you say to patients as what you do to them. An early, frank admission of a mistake, or sorrow expressed for a bad outcome, may deflect, or obviate, more serious difficulties later.

My philosophy boils down to Stoicism, Samaritanism and Love. The first two principles I have discussed already. The last is far more difficult to define and quantify. What is it then? It seems to me to be a complex mixture of physical attraction, caring and friendship, with one or other of these emotions predominating at the different ages, stages and scenes of life. I am reminded of Whitsun Week in Manchester and the Church parades (Chapter 3). The children used to carry large banners with the emblem 'God is Love' picked out in flowers. Some years ago, Sir James Black suggested to me that we should turn this statement on its head and say rather that 'Love is God'. I think that this is a valuable insight and draws together caring, charity and Samaritanism.

For more than forty years my wife Judith has been my lover, nurse, companion and friend. When we were married in 1960 we barely knew each other, but it proved to be an inspired choice. At first we were sustained by physical passion; as time has gone we have been tempered in the crucible of illness and loss. I can therefore say with the writer of Ecclesiastes that, 'Blessed is the man that hath a virtuous wife, for his days shall be double'. Robert Southey, the Lakeland Poet, has also summarized these feelings I now have, far better than I could ever do, in his magnificent poem The Curse of Kehama:-

> They sin who tell us Love can die
> With life all other passions fly,
> All others are but vanity.
> In heaven Ambition cannot dwell,
> Nor Avarice in the Vaults of Hell;
> Earthly these passions of the earth,
> They perish where they had their birth
> But love is indestructible'.

In this short biography, I have tried, however inadequately, to summarize my voyage through a life in medicine. Like Odysseus, I have faced storms, trials and setbacks. For a greater part of the time it has, despite all these difficulties, been highly enjoyable and rewarding. When it ceased to be fulfilling I stopped doing it.

One of my research fellows, over a beer in Leeds, once asked me what I would like to see as my epitaph. For a time this question stumped me. Eventually after considerable thought (and several more beers) I came up with the statement, 'He did what he could'. I will, on reflection, settle for that!

Bibliography

Chapters 1 & 2
A Child's War: Growing Up on the Home Front. 2000
Author: Mike Brown
Sutton Publishing, Stroud, Gloucestershire
ISBN 0-7509-2441-1

Chapter 3
Harrison's Principles of Internal Medicine. Twelfth Edition. 1991
Pages 933-938. Rheumatic fever.
Page 1526. Pernicious anaemia.
McGraw-Hill Inc. Publishers, New York
ISBN 0-079749-8.

Chapter 4
Wesley: His Own Biographer. 1896
Selections from the Journals of the Reverend John Wesley. Sometime
Fellow of Lincoln College, Oxford.
Publisher; C.E. Kelly, London.

The Oxygen of Ignorance. 2002
Author: Thomson, Bob
The Scottish Review. Volume 2. Number 4. pp.1-4.
This is an essay on the divisive and damaging nature of religious schools.

Chapter 5
Bogota Bandit: The Outlaw Life of Charlie Mitten. 1996
Author: Richard Adamson
Publishers: Mainstream, Edinburgh
ISBN 1-85158-867-1.

Winners and Champions: The Story of Manchester United's 1948 FA Cup and 1952 Championship Winning Teams. 1985
Author: Alec Shorrocks
Publishers: Arthur Baker Ltd, London
ISBN 0-213-16920-7

Lancashire: A History of County Cricket. 1972
Author: John Kay
Publishers: Arthur Barker Ltd, London
ISBN 0-213-16405-1

Chapter 6
Richard Cobden: A Victorian Outsider. 1987
Author: Wendy Hinde
Publishers: Yale University Press: New Haven and London
ISBN 0-300-03880-1

Chapter 7
The Manchester Grammar School: 1515-1915.
Author: Alfred A. Mumford. 1919.
Publisher: Longmans, Green & Co., 39 Paternoster Row, London.

James, Eric John Francis.
1909-1992. Lord James of Rusholme.
Obituary: The Times. Tuesday May 19, 1992. Page 15.

Chapter 8
The Secession to Stamford.
Brasenose Quatercentenary Monographs. 1909. Vol. II pp. 15-20.
The Northern Faction of Monks shows independence of mind; tenacity and resilience.
They decamp to Lincolnshire.

Chapter 9
The Owens College: Its Foundation and Growth. 1886
Author: Joseph Thompson.
Publisher: J.E. Cornish, Manchester.

Portrait of a University. 1851-1951.
Author: D.G. Charlton. 1951.
Publisher: Manchester University Press, Manchester.

Chapter 10
In Time of Need: A History of the Royal Lancaster Infirmary.
Author: John G. Blacktop.
Published privately in Lancaster in the 1990s. A copy is held in the
Lancaster Reference Library.

Chapter 11
Portrait of a Hospital. 1752-1948.
To commemorate the bicentenary of the Manchester Royal Infirmary.
Author: W. Brockbank. 1952.
Publisher: Heinemann, London.

Professor Sir Douglas Black. 1913-2002.
Doctor who led the BMA and the Royal College.
Daily Telegraph Obituary 2002.
September 16th.
See Also Brit. Med. J. *325* 661-662.

Chapter 12
Cochrane, Archibald Leman. (1909-1988).
Munk's Roll of the Royal College of Physicians of London. Pp. 95-97.

**One Man's Medicine: An Autobiography of Professor Archie
Cochrane.** 1989
Authors: A.L. Cochrane and M. Blythe.
Publishers: Memoir Club.
ISBN 0-7279-0277.

Chapter 13
Peart W.S. 1970
Death of the Professor of Medicine.
Lancet I pp. 401-402.

Peart W.S. 1983
Rebirth of the Professor of Medicine.
Lancet I pp. 810-812.

Chapter 14
Pickering, Sir George White. 1904-1980.
Obituary. Munk's Roll of the Royal College of Physicians, London.
Volume VII pp. 464-467.

Lee, M.R. 1965
The estimation of renin in biological fluids.
Thesis for the Degree of Doctor of Philosophy; Oxford University.

Robertson, P.W., Klidjian, A., Harding, L.K., Walters, G., Lee, M.R. and Robb-Smith, A.H.T. 1967
Hypertension due to a renin-secreting tumour.
Amer. J. Med. *43* 963-976.

Chapter 15
Martin Luther King: A Critical Biography. 1970
Author: David L. Lewis.
Publishers: Allen Lane, London.
ISBN 0713-9005-39.

Fundamental and Applied Research Aids in the Synthesis of a Thyroid Hormone. 1968
The Record of the National Institutes of Health; Bethesda; Maryland, U.S.A.
Volume XX Number 11.

Chapter 16
Renin and Hypertension: A Modern Synthesis. 1969
Author: M.R. Lee.
Publisher: Lloyd-Luke; 49 Newman Street, London.

Chapter 17
Dowling, R.H. 1983
Cholelithiasis: Medical Treatment.
Clinics in Gastroenterology *12* 125-178.

Chapter 18
A History of the Leeds School of Medicine: One and a Half Centuries (1831-1981). 1982
Authors: Anning, S.T. and Walls, W.K.J.
Publisher: Leeds University Press.

C.J. Lote. Advances in Renal Physiology. 1986
Chapter 7. Dopamine and the Kidney by M.R. Lee pp. 218-246.
Publisher: Croom Helm Ltd., Kent BR3 1AT.
ISBN 0-7099-1682-5.

Chapter 19
The Royal Infirmary of Edinburgh: Bicentenary Year 1729-1929.
Author: A. Logan Turner 1929.
Publisher: Oliver and Boyd, Tweeddale Court, Edinburgh.

Fellows of Edinburgh's College of Physicians During the Scottish Enlightenment. 2001
Author: Reginald Passmore.
Publisher: Royal College of Physicians, Edinburgh.
ISBN 0-85405-057-4.

Chapter 20
Death's Doings 1826.
Author: Richard Dagley.
Death and the Cricketer by Barnard Batwell pp. 53-56.
Publisher: Andrews and Cole, London.

Chapter 21
The King James Bible. (Revised Authorised Version)
The Gospel according to Saint Luke; Chapter 10; Verses 29 to 37.
The Parable of the Good Samaritan.

Douglas, A. 1984
Promises to Keep. Presidential Address to the British Thoracic Society.
Thorax *39* 481–486.

McCormick, J. 1979
The doctor: father-figure or plumber.
Publisher: Croom Helm Ltd. (see above).

McDermott, W. and Rogers, D.E. 1983
Technology's Consort.
Amer. J. Med *74* 353–358.

Pickering, G.W. 1964
Physician and Scientist: Harveian Oration to the Royal College of
Physicians in London.
Brit. Med. J. *ii* 1615–1619.

Index

Note: MRL denotes the author Michael Radcliffe Lee.